In N

An Unlikely Runner's Guide to Running ...and Life

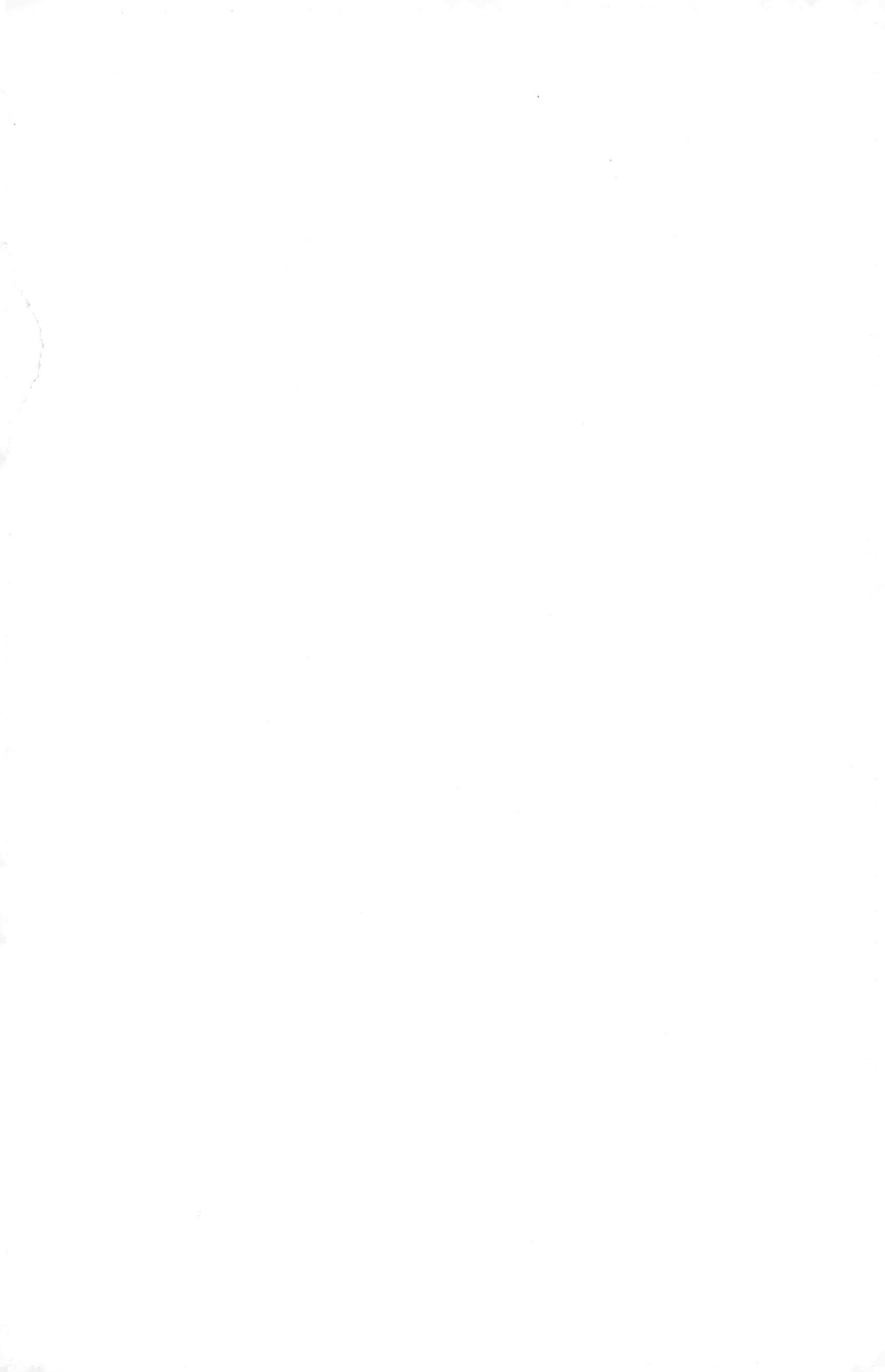

In My Shoes:

An Unlikely Runner's Guide to Running ...and Life

Josh Wackler

In My Shoes:

An Unlikely Runner's Guide to Running ...and Life

© 2019 by Josh Wackler. All Rights Reserved.

Published by Wackler Enterprise

Cover by Sweet 'N Spicy Designs (http://sweetnspicydesigns.com)
Edited by Barbara Ardinger

All rights reserved. No parts of this book may be reproduced or transmitted in any form without written permission from the publisher, except by reviewers who may quote brief excerpts in connection with a review.

The miracle isn't that I finished. The miracle is that I had the courage to start.

—John Bingham

Acknowledgement

I want to thank the members of my review team, the people who read this book as a work in progress. Thanks to:

1) Damian Barreiro
2) Meg Belcher
3) Dr. Kimberly Brengle
4) Laurie Kamerer
5) Dr. Audra Lance
6) Dr. Callie Lance

Thanks also to my editor, Barbara Ardinger, Ph.D., who turned my "regular guy" writing into the better prose you've read in this book. Thanks also to Sue Jorgenson, who proofread the finished manuscript, and to Eileen Troemel, who helped me find a cover designer, gave me excellent advice about publishing this book and assisted with self-publishing.

Contents

Foreword

Preface Why Am I Writing This Book?

1 Follow Your Heart 1
Appendix to Chapter 1 5
2 Be Humble 9
3 Failure Is Inevitable 19
4 It's Heart That Matters 25
5 Be Patient 34
6 Running Is Cheaper than Therapy 42
7 Differences vs. Faults 48
Appendix to Chapter 7 54
8 Pay It Forward 60
9 Be a Better Person 68
10 Destination vs. Journey 72
11 Slow Down to Go Faster 78
12 Motivation 82
13 Dream Big 88
14 Stop Complaining 91
15 Questions Beginning Runners Often Ask 95
16 Unwritten Rules 107

Foreword

If you'd asked me ten years ago what kind of book my brother might one day write, here's what I would have said: "Josh could write a book about hunting or fishing or bartending. Definitely about leadership or customer service. No, wait—this will be his first book: *101 Reasons I Will Never Be a Runner*."

Sure, Josh had done his share of running all his life. Mostly on sports teams and when being chased by a bear. For years he marveled at my running marathon after marathon and staying in "marathon shape" as a lifestyle. As a working mother of young children, I discovered running with friends as a clever way to try to maintain a social life. To Josh, however, this was in the "two wrongs don't make a right" school of thought: running sucks and having a standing 5:30 a.m. appointment to run also sucks.

That's why, at first, I didn't pay much attention when he started making the occasional inquiry about running. What kind of shoes do you wear? Are the shoes that important? Is the "runner's high" really a thing? Do you eat before you run?

Before I knew it, Josh had run a half marathon. And then another. And another, in which he took second place. He clearly had the speed to qualify for the Boston Marathon. And he also clearly had his sights set on that very goal. For many runners, qualifying for Boston is the Holy Grail of running. Most find it an epic feat. But Josh has a secret weapon: he is very, *very* stubborn.

He qualified for Boston in his second marathon. In contrast, I'd run a dozen marathons—including his qualifying race—before I managed my own qualifying time. And only then with the help of a highly motivational pacer: my brother.

Josh started running races as an experiment. First to see if he could run 13.1. Then to see if he could run 26.2. And finally to see if he could run 26.2 in a ridiculously stingy amount of time. By the time he stood at the starting line of the Boston Marathon in Hopkinton (just outside Boston) in 2012, running had come to mean so much more to him. Community. Comradery. The joy of helping others find their own starting line…and the wonder of watching them cross the finish line. The profound strength of the human spirit.

As it turns out, his first book is called *In My Shoes: An Unlikely Runner's Guide to Running...and Life.*

—Laurie Kamerer

Preface:

Why Am I Writing This Book?

I'm the last person who should write a book about running. In fact, if I had told my twenty-five-year old self that one day I would be writing a book about running, that self would have my current self committed.

So why am I actually writing this book? There are numerous books on running already out there, and if mine isn't any different than those books, then what's the point of writing a new one? It's a question I have struggled with for years, mostly because I don't closely resemble anybody who has written any running book I have ever seen.

I didn't run in college or in the Olympics for Bill Bowerman, the American track and field coach and co-founder of Nike, Inc. (See Kenny Moore, Bowerman and the Men of Oregon: The Story of Oregon's Legendary Coach and Nike's Cofounder (Rodale Books, 2007).) I'm not sponsored by Asics, Clif, or Garmin. I have never run fifty marathons in fifty states in fifty days. I've never run an ultra, or a 50k race. (See Dean Karnazes, *50/50: Secrets I Learned Running 50 Marathons in 50 Days—and How You Too Can Achieve Super Endurance!* (Grand Central Life & Style, 2009).)

Nor am I part of a running tribe in Mexico. (See Christopher McDougall, *Born to Run: A Hidden Tribe, Superathletes, and the Greatest Race the World Has Never Seen* (Vintage, 2011).) I've never won a gold medal. I have all of my arms and legs and am in pretty good health. I'm not dying from cancer. I am not a senior writer for *Sports Illustrated* and I can't run a marathon in 2:10 or a mile in four minutes. At 6'7", 245 pounds, I more closely resemble a power forward than a runner, and I have often been told all the reasons why I cannot and should not run because of my body type. I grew up playing, following, and admiring the traditional American sports of basketball, baseball, and football. Not running. In fact, I hated running while I was growing up.

In a traditional sense, and compared to other books about running, I have absolutely no business writing such a book. So you might ask, why am I writing this book?

After much deliberation and blogging about running, it finally hit me. My hesitation to write a book arises from my lack of status as a traditional runner and writer. Which is exactly the reason why I felt compelled to write this book. All those reasons listed above, all the things that I am not and have not done…they're exactly the reasons that compelled me to begin writing.

We "normal" folks need a voice.

I'm a normal person with a normal job, just like you. While I have thoroughly enjoyed every running book I've ever read, each for different reasons, I find that I sometimes have a difficult time relating to the author and his/her story. I have always wanted to hear from the perspective of a "normal" runner. One who has never been a professional writer. Who learns about running through his own mistakes rather than from a professional coach. Who must navigate his daily work schedule to fit running in despite a hectic schedule. Who has to squeeze money out of an already tight budget for travel and registration costs to run in races, since those costs are not covered by some other means. Someone I have never heard of in *Runner's World*.

Ultimately, my hope is to show anyone and everyone that, with the exception of very few folks, *anyone can be a runner*. You don't have to have a certain body type or background or status. Yes, there are certain clubs and societies in the world that are exclusive and that some of us can't get into. You have to belong. But the roads…the roads are always open.

Running is a very simple act, one we are all genetically ingrained with the ability to do, provided we make the effort. You lace up your shoes and go running until you decide to stop. That's it.

But we try to make it complicated and come up with all sorts of nonsensical reasons why we cannot or should not run. But that's exactly what most of those reasons are. *Nonsensical*.

Through my years of running and training for marathons, I continue to be thoroughly amazed at how much something so simple has taught me about life in general. Lessons in running parallel lessons in life. And I feel compelled to share those lessons with you and other readers of my book.

I should point out two key facts you should remember as you read the following pages to make sure I'm not giving you the wrong impression. First, I am not a doctor, nor do I have any education in health or medicine. Anything I write about related to injuries, treatment, or health in general should be taken with that in mind.

Second, everybody—and every body—is different. What works or doesn't work for me is going to be different from what works for just about any other person. Don't always take what I write as fact. I'm writing about what I have observed through my own trials and errors.

Please keep these two points in mind as you decide what's best for you and your body.

There are a few other matters that are important for me to spell out. I am not perfect. I have never been perfect, I will never be perfect, and I will never claim to be perfect. When I refer to lessons I have learned and words of wisdom I have come to try and live by, please note that, just like anyone else, I can fall short of those lessons and that wisdom on a daily basis. I simply try hard every day to do the best I can to live up to them.

Throughout the following pages you'll notice suggestions of the type of household I grew up in. We weren't the type of family that talked in depth about our feelings, and we certainly weren't the type of family to go to a counselor or attend therapy. What did I learn growing up? You deal with life as it happens, take it in stride, and find your own ways to cope with whatever you're dealing with. And if you fail? Good. Welcome to the real world. Deal with it.

Unless something was obviously broken or we couldn't get out of bed, we didn't go to the doctor. My parents had a "you'll be fine" approach. They were also adamant about our doing things "the right way." For example, if you're going to go play on the baseball team, you're not going to do it half-assed. You'll do it right and work harder and pour more heart into it than anyone else. If not, you won't be playing at all.

Unbeknownst to me, all those childhood lessons and beliefs became the foundation to exactly how I approach my running. They're how I still approach life. It certainly shows in the following chapters.

But we'll get to all that.

Am I looking for wealth or fame? Notoriety or recognition? A new job as a writer at some fancy newspaper or magazine? Hardly. My motivation for writing this book is as simple as having a mindset that running is a simple act.

I'm writing for inspiration. Not inspiration for myself, but for you. If I pour hundreds of hours into these pages and soak them with my blood, sweat, and tears, and through it all I don't make a dime or gain an ounce of fame, that's okay. But if I inspire just one person to take up running, it's worth it to me.

Inspiring other people to be better is an amazing feeling. One of the best. Which was another lesson taught to me by running when I coached my first trainee for their first race.

But we'll get to that also.

I hope you enjoy the following stories even just a fraction as much as I enjoyed living through them.

Happy reading. And happy running.

1

Follow Your Heart

The 2013 Boston Marathon bombing reverberated around the world. Like so many horrendous acts in history, it was an attack on a sacred institution. For runners, it was a kick in the stomach that continues to ache and will forever ache.

There are no words I can use to describe the spectrum of emotions that hit me when my phone rang on April 15, 2013. A friend was calling to make sure I wasn't running in Boston that year. He wanted to find out if I was safe, but when I asked why, the other end of the phone went silent. He didn't know how to tell me. All he could say was "Turn the news on."

So I turned on the news. My heart sank. Fear. Sadness. Confusion. And anger.

You have no idea how angry I was. How angry I still am.

I will write on the following pages about how special the Boston Marathon is. How life affirming the experience is. But "special" and "life-affirming" are not strong enough. The Boston Marathon is a magical event that accomplishes something rare in the world today: this race unites not just a city, but people around the world, in a shared passion and a shared sense of humanity. For this one day, there are no divisions along political lines. No divisions among religion. Nobody sees racial differences or any of the other identity markers we wage war over. There is only this: *the love of running and of those who run.*

So you can imagine my utter disbelief that someone would do something so heinous to try to ruin the marathon.

I also felt fortunate, as my sister and I had the bombing surrounded, so to speak. I ran Boston in 2012, the bombing was 2013, she ran it in 2014, I ran it again in 2015, and she logged her second race in 2016. Somehow we were fortunate enough to have been out of harm's way.

Other runners, volunteers, and spectators, unfortunately, were not so lucky. People lost arms. Feet. Legs. Some even lost their lives. There was such a profound emotional response that when beloved Boston Red Sox designated hitter David Ortiz said in a pregame speech at Fenway Park on national TV, "This is our fucking city. And nobody is going to dictate our freedom," nobody seemed bothered by the public F-bomb. The FCC had a chance to discipline Ortiz and others involved in the broadcast. They chose not to. This situation gave Mr. Ortiz a Mulligan, a free shot, so to speak. Rightfully so.

We Boston Marathon runners are in our own sort of fraternity. Once you've run Boston, you're a member of an unofficial club of brothers and sisters. So when this tragedy struck the Marathon and nearly every American citizen felt the sting, we Boston alumni felt a worse sting. Our family was under attack. We'd done nothing to deserve that attack. Some of those runners will never run again, which is tragic to a level that is difficult to explain to a non-runner.

When I registered to run Boston for the second time in 2015, I was shocked at the number of people in my life who called to ask me not to run it. They kept insisting that I should withdraw. Well, yes, I thought about it. But not for long. I was running the Boston Marathon. Safety be damned.

Here's why. If I change my mind about running, my decisions, my actions, and my life would be based on an act of terror. Then I would be letting those terrorists win. That was exactly what those two brothers were trying to accomplish. And I'll be damned, I said, if I let them succeed.

Post-bombing, the race changed. The next year, there were SWAT, National Guard, and military personnel everywhere, ten times more than I remembered from 2012. Security at the runners' village near the start was significantly tighter. Sniffing dogs were everywhere.

But do you know what didn't change? The citizens of Boston. In fact, I would argue that the support the year after the bombing was at a higher level than ever before.

And so I say: Hats off to the citizens of Boston. And to the city of Boston in general. They could have run away. They could have gone and hidden in the shadows. When they got punched in the gut and brought to their knees, they could have waved the white flag. Instead, they got right back up. With tears in their eyes and blood dripping from their noses, they looked terror right in the face and told it they would not be bullied. Bostonians could have buckled, but they chose to hit back. They were—and are—tenacious.

Runners showed similar toughness. In the immediate aftermath of the bombing, hundreds of sore and weary runners stood in line to give blood. I can assure you that after you've run 26.2 miles, you have no desire to even walk down the block, much less stand in line and donate an entire pint of your blood. But there's this truth about runners: we have a high tolerance for discomfort and a universal sense of brotherhood. People needed help and the runners that day were helping in the only way they knew how.

Thank you to the people and to the runners of Boston. You taught us a lesson in life. A lesson that I, for one, will never forget.

I'm glad that—in returning—I did my small part. Was there a part of my brain that was questioning my actions? Of course there was. It was in the back of everybody's mind. But I never really entertained the idea of dropping out. My heart and my head were both telling me that going through with it was the right thing to do. And when I listen to my heart and my conscience, they never lead me down the wrong path.

Jiminy Cricket was right. "Let your conscience be your guide."

Life lesson learned: *Follow your heart.*

Appendix to Chapter 1

I asked my sister to share some of her perspective as a Boston runner the first year after the bomb. The following is her perspective:

2014: The Year We Took Our Race Back

By Laurie Kamerer

It was April 15, 2013, and I was hard at work in my office when I started receiving frantic texts from friends and family:
Status?
Please let me know you are safe.
Are you in Boston?
Where are you?

My heart sank. I dashed off quick replies, googled news about the Boston Marathon, and joined the world in utter devastation and despair. Someone had exploded bombs at the race. But almost instantly, devastation and despair were joined by a third—more powerful—emotion. Defiance.

Several months earlier, I'd finally snagged my first Boston Qualifying time. Although the loved ones who'd texted me after the bombing were assuming that I was running Boston 2013, in fact, I'd qualified for Boston 2014 and would race then, terrorism be damned, because here's something everyone should know about marathoners: we are some of the grittiest motherfuckers you will ever meet.

While every runner has his or her own unique motivation for logging miles, my non-scientific studies suggest that fitness is not the most common motivation. Some of us are running away from our demons. Others are self-medicating for anxiety, sadness, or stress. Many people use running as a social outlet or to find a sense of community.

Having one or more of these motives makes it easier to withstand the rigors of marathon training, which comes with no shortage of inconveniences. Boatloads of stinky laundry. Injuries. Blisters. Barfing. Chafing. Lost toenails. Menacing dogs, cars, even other people. Emergency diarrhea with no bathrooms in sight. And the excruciating pain upon hitting the proverbial wall. That's just a few.

But the joy of racing in a marathon eclipses all of the above. Nowhere is this more true than at the Boston Marathon. My heart raced with anticipation 367 days after the bombing as I walked toward the starting line at Hopkinton. Security was tight, and I made a point of thanking every member of the military and police force I passed along the way. Waiting for the starting gun, I mentally ticked through my usual disciplined race plan: *pace, efficiency, hydration, nutrition*.

The gun went off. And my plans went out the window. Here's the thing about the Boston Marathon: it's the only sporting event in the world where an average person is treated like a superstar. From start to finish, the course is lined with spectators, sometimes five people deep on both sides of the road. The spectators are there not just to cheer a friend or family member. It's the people of Boston hosting a party for the world. And they know how to host. And they stay all day.

In 2014, the Boston Marathon attendance set an all-time record. Cheering was just the start of it. Many fans were holding signs:

1) *Today we remember. Today we run.*
2) *We "AH" Boston strong.*
3) *This parade sucks. (a perennial favorite of mine)*
4) *Kiss me. (at Wellesley College)*

Other fans handed out water, gummy bears, pretzels, Oreos, oranges, bananas, red licorice, coffee, popsicles, pickles…you name it, they had it for us. Kids held their hands out for high fives.

I forgot to drink water, but I indulged in everything else. I zig-zagged back and forth to high-five people. I eagerly accepted snacks from every stranger. It was like I thought the sport was "marathon smorgasbording." I cheered for every guide runner as well as the people they were enabling to run the race.

I wasn't alone in this revelry, of course. I've never been so sure that everyone was united around a common cause, that we were enveloped in a sense of universal humanity. Nobody talked about religion or politics. If someone tripped, people rushed to help them up.

That was the day we took the Boston Marathon back, and the fair citizens of Boston came out with plenty of signs to thank us for doing so.

2

Be Humble

I'm a guy. A prototypical guy. Paint a picture of a stereotypical young male, and you'll get something that fairly closely resembles me. I'm a football fanatic. I love beer and pizza. I'll pay hundreds of dollars for a ticket to certain sporting events but you couldn't pay me a thousand dollars to be seen at the ballet. I once had a "man cave" in my house with painted walls showing my three beloved sports teams, the Pittsburgh Steelers, the St. Louis Cardinals, and the Oregon State Beavers. But I'm married now, so the "man cave" is obviously not a reality anymore.

I grew up playing traditional sports. I drive a pickup and like to hunt and fish. And just like most guys I have ever met, I have pride. Quite a bit of pride. Maybe too much at times.

Ego and hubris are common maladies among us guys. Which makes sense, I suppose, when you think about the genetics of us and our fellow mammals. Having some background in biology, I know that deep down inside, we mammals have two basic priorities in our lives: survival and reproduction. Our sophisticated human brains are constantly processing thoughts of survival and reproduction. When you break it down to the basics, those are the two priorities our brains historically evolved to focus on.

With our omnipresent wisdom (insert sarcastic tone here), we guys often think that the more we talk and brag about our accomplishments, about how cool we are—like my story/truck/life being more interesting/bigger/cooler than yours—the more likely chance we'll have at reproduction. The irony here is how easily we can be annoyed at others for their chest-beating but turn around seconds later and do the same thing in an effort to one-up them.

We all know the type. The "one-up guy" who, any time you tell a story about anything, is sure to one-up you with his story, which relates to yours but is somehow just slightly better. Have you ever listened to a conversation between two one-up guys? It's as mind numbing as watching Roger Federer in a tennis match against a cement wall. But as annoyed as we get when we notice other people doing that, at some point in our lives, we are all guilty of it.

Running has taught me this lesson in its own clever way.

I was at a conference in Washington, D.C., awhile back and got up one morning to get a run in. I jumped at the opportunity to run past as many monuments as possible. I was amazed at how many sites and buildings I was able to see in one forty-five-minute run.

At one point I turned right to head toward the World War II Memorial. Upon arrival, I tried to make a left turn to run in front of it, but the narrow sidewalk was being completely blocked by two older men. I was instantly annoyed. This is a sidewalk, I said to myself. How inconsiderate and discourteous these old dudes are to block my path! I'd like you to get out of my way and apologize this instant.

But then I looked closer. They were both in wheelchairs and were being pushed by men who were probably in their mid-fifties. One could presume that it was a pair of father and sons. Access to the sidewalk was being blocked by their wheelchairs not because they were being intentionally discourteous but because they had paused to gaze at the wonderment of the Memorial. Upon closer look they were both wearing *USS Missouri* hats named for a battleship used heavily during World War II.

These old men were veterans. World War II veterans at that.

Being inconsiderate was no doubt the last thing on the minds of these gentlemen. They were simply appreciating the moment. The moment they may have been waiting decades for. To stare in wonderment at the Memorial they had helped create by serving this great country.

My shoulders sank, and I suddenly felt like I was the size of the ant I saw scurrying along the sidewalk. Not ten seconds ago, I was convinced that my run—my training—was a bigger priority than anything anyone around these monuments could be doing. And how dare they impede me in my important task.

I turned to gaze at the monument with them. To this day, I have no comprehension of what must have been going through their heads because I also have no comprehension what they went through during their service in the war. But one thing I can say for sure is that all my impatience for the situation was gone in an instant. I stood there for a long time, with a metaphorical lump in my throat and foot in my mouth, allowing the four gentlemen as much time as they wanted.

It's safe to say they had earned that right.

Sometimes it's hard for us to remember that the world doesn't revolve around us. What's important to us and what our priorities are don't necessarily dictate the priorities of other people. And just because we have accomplished something and we've done it bigger or faster or more often than someone else, that doesn't mean that it's any better than anyone else's accomplishment. It's just different.

Yet another life lesson running has taught me.

When I ran my first race, the Hospital Hill Half Marathon in June 2008 in Kansas City, Missouri, I was beaming with pride. Ten weeks prior to that race, I had never run more than three miles in my entire life. But I'd signed up for it, and I ran it in a respectable time, despite having a mild case of bronchitis and a nagging IT Band problem. (At the time, I had no clue it was an IT Band issue—I just knew the outside of my knee was on fire). I thought I was pretty cool, and I was set on telling people how cool I was because of how fast I'd run despite all of those circumstances working against me.

I finished in the top twenty percent of all finishers, I said to my imaginary audience, so I must be cooler and a better runner than eighty percent of the people out there. And in my first race, no less!

What a jackass I was.

I was assuming people thought I was cooler simply because I was running faster, and I was judging people based on the fact that they ran slower than me.

But don't ever let anyone judge you in your running. Ever. Unless you're being blatantly lazy. People sometimes tell me how they wish running were as easy for them as it is for me. They tell me how lucky I am to be blessed with such talent.

Easy? Running is not easy. Not for anyone. Not even the elites. They have their bad days just like you and me. They get their asses kicked, too. They have moments of doubt. They have injuries. They have heartbreak. They have mornings when they wake up and just don't feel like running.

Every runner does.

Many people don't have the luxury of seeing what other runners go through. What I go through. They either forget or don't realize that after half of all of my long runs (15+ miles), I puke. That I sit on the couch feeling like death. That my body is in so much shock I can't stop shivering. That I can't navigate stairs. That when I hop into the shower the next morning, I have to stop myself from screaming because of the chafing on certain parts of my body. That I sometimes wear a golf ball-sized blood blister on the inside of my right foot. That after one race, it was so hot I lost over an inch on my waistline due to all the fluid depletion and came within a second away from passing out in the finish area.

When I first started running races and my times kept improving, I developed an ego. I thought I was somehow better than most runners simply because my times were better. I believed my superiority was inevitable, and that I obviously worked harder than those people. The proof was that I run faster.

The irony here is that I was making the same mistake as those folks who thought running was easy for me. The more I run, the more I learn that running is hard for everyone. From the one-milers to the elite professionals, running is challenging. It always will be.

I would, in fact, argue that the people who work the hardest during a race—and who have the most heart—are the people with the slowest times. I have a tremendous amount of respect for those people.

Most races have luxuries set up for us runners, like aid stations with water and food, crowd support, traffic control, an announcer and music, and a finish area complete with amenities. But after five or six hours, most marathons open up the course and start tearing things down. So those folks who run their race in over six hours are essentially left to fend for themselves. No more aid stations. No more people cheering them on (which makes a bigger difference than any non-runner will ever realize). No more traffic control. No more finish line.

Those six-hour-plus runners choose to continue running without water, having to dodge traffic, wondering if there will be anyone left at the finish line, or even if they'll be awarded an official finishing time. They are fueled solely by desire. Desire to keep running, no matter what. By the time they cross the finish line, most of the other runners have already showered, eaten a good hot meal, and are probably celebrating with friends (and fans) over a tall, frosty beverage.

Once upon a time I thought the six-hour-plus runners were half-assing the marathon. I thought they just didn't have any heart. My regular-guy ego was dominating my viewpoint. I was, so to speak, running on hubris. But the opposite is actually true. I have now changed my mind. I understand that those folks have more heart and more desire to finish than I've ever had. And I have the utmost respect for them and the grit they show.

Logic forces us to conclude that the more races a runner completes and the faster their time gets, the more egotistical they become about their own running because they have more accomplishments to brag about. Interestingly enough, the opposite tends to be true. The more I run, the more I realize I don't like the people who brag about their accomplishments or put other runners down because they haven't run as far or as fast.

After that first race, I see now, I was mistaken to think that I was better than eighty percent of the other runners. I merely crossed the finish line at a different time than they did. Nothing more, nothing less.

But my egotistical thoughts didn't die. They still pop up from time to time, no matter how hard I try to stamp that hubris out.

I even used to cite my size as an excuse to suggest how much better a runner I would be if my body type were a little bit different. I'm the size of a football player and certainly don't fit the mold of a runner. I used to be very quick to point out how fast my times were "for a guy my size." But I eventually gave that excuse up because it was exactly that: an excuse.

Rather than owning up to their own actions or lack thereof, people tend to come up with creative excuses. That drives me crazy, so I made a conscious decision a few years ago to completely remove my own excuse from my conversations. I'm not "pretty fast for a guy my size." My times and distances are my times and distances. Period. And whatever my times and distances are, they're more than acceptable. I don't need the disclaimer about "my size" because the only purpose the disclaimer ever served was to fuel my ego. My ego has never needed fueling.

Those lessons have spilled over into real life in almost every facet you can think of. Nobody likes an egotistical guy. Not in their family, in their professional life, in their hobbies or other sports. It drives us nuts when someone obviously thinks too highly of themselves and thinks they're better than the people around them.

Remember when Lebron James left Cleveland and announced he was going to take his talents to South Beach? He did this on a nationally televised "look how cool I am" ESPN special. The world outside of Miami was revolted.

When you're at a restaurant or a bar, nobody likes a bad tipper because it almost seems like a sign from the customer to the wait staff that they are somehow better than those staff members.

Have you ever had a condescending boss? It makes your job and your life miserable. Because you know in your heart of hearts that your boss isn't necessarily better than you. They just happen to have a different role in the company.

On the other hand we admire athletes who shed the limelight and stick to working hard towards their goals, we praise people who tip well and treat their wait staff like they are actual people and we yearn for bosses who praise us and make sure we understand that we are just as important to the team as they are.

You won't hear many long-time runners who have above-average times bragging about their accomplishments. That's because running has taught them to praise the good work of others instead of their own work. It's something we learn over miles and miles on the pavement.

Another lesson that takes some of us longer to learn than others has to do with how swiftly we cover our distances. Ask any long-time runner and, except for the elites who are competing for big dollars and Boston championships, almost every single experienced runner will agree to this: *pace is overrated.*

I preached this idea for a long time before I truly got a grasp on it, but now every single part of me knows that it's true. It took an apparent near-death experience for me to fully get it.

My first Boston Marathon was on April 16, 2012. I had been preparing for and trying to run this race for years, and when I actually stood at the starting line, my excitement level was sky high. My training had gone extremely well, and I was ready to PR with a sub 2:50 finish time at the world's most prestigious race. To put that into perspective, that would mean a 6:39/mile average pace.

But the weather had other plans for the race. It was eighty-seven degrees in Boston on that day, the second hottest day in the race's history. Although there were 5,000 registrants who elected to not run the race, of the 20,000 that still participated, over 2,100 received medical treatment due to dehydration and heat exhaustion. Many more than that, myself included, probably should have received medical treatment. While eighty-seven doesn't seem scorching hot, it's important to remember that most runners that day had done their peak training during the months of January, February, and March. Over ninety percent of my training runs were done in temperatures below forty degrees. Our bodies just weren't ready for that kind of hot weather.

But I was bound and determined to still run a fast time despite the heat. I ran my first five miles in thirty-six minutes. But when I noticed I was starting to get the chills and had goose bumps all over my body, I had my come-to-Jesus moment. My great insight. I said to myself, "You can either be hauled away today in an ambulance or you can swallow some of your pride and cross the finish line under your own power. It's your choice."

I was running in Boston. THE Boston Marathon. I was already there, already qualified. What, exactly, did I have to prove to anyone? Why did it matter whether I ran that race in under two and a half or over five hours? I had received dozens of phone calls, texts, emails, and Facebook messages from friends and family all over the country who congratulated me, wished me luck and, above all, told me to be safe.

Guess how many of them mentioned how fast I should run? Not one. No one cared about my pace.

I was amazed at how my perspective changed when I swallowed my pride. Typically, I am very focused in a race. Focused on my pace, focused on my time, focused on how I'm feeling, focused on how the rest of the race is going to go. But when I let go of worrying about my pace, it was an epiphany.

My entire approach to the race changed. I started handing out high fives to every little kid and every military, police, and fire personnel standing along the course. I said thank you to all those personnel for everything they do to protect us. I also developed an enormous appreciation for the Boston crowd, not just because there were so many of them along the route, but because of the zest and enthusiasm they showed in cheering us runners on.

When I crossed the finish line in a mortal (well, actually, average) time of 4:20, eighty-one minutes slower than my qualifying time, every single volunteer in the finish area made it a point to congratulate and thank every runner, including me, just for participating. I had random citizens of Boston doing the same thing the entire three and a half days I was there. As I was hobbling along a sidewalk with my dad after the race, I even met a family of strangers who gave me a standing ovation. Dad and I were both fighting back tears. And of course Dad kept stopping to brag that his son had just finished the Boston Marathon.

"They know, Dad," I whispered. "They know."

Yes, it was a special day, and it took something that special for it to fully click in my head that pace is in fact overrated. I had preached that idea for years, and while I thought I understood it, I didn't have a full comprehension until that scorching Monday morning. It's so simple, yet so difficult for people to gain an understanding, mostly because of pride. Which was what had been holding me back.

Did 10,000 people finish ahead of me? Yes, they did. But that doesn't mean any of them had a better experience than I did. They simply crossed the finish line at a different time of the day. Ego was the only reason why their times might have mattered. I made the decision mid-race to let go of that ego.

A marathon is an experience. Not a race. And Boston is the pinnacle experience. My pace that day was by far the slowest I have ever run a marathon. But I had by far the best experience I have ever had in a marathon. But the pre-Boston version of Josh Wackler would have laughed in your face if you had tried to convince him that was even possible.

After hobbling through the finish area and finding the family waiting area, I found a place to sit down. My sore, aching feet and legs were grateful to relax and not be moving. It took my family and friends a while to find me, so I had some time to reflect on the marathon and how much it didn't go the way I had it all planned out in my head. I wondered for a moment if my friends or family would be disappointed in my time.

What a silly thought.

I finished the marathon ninety minutes slower than I had hoped. Which was disappointing, no doubt. But on the other hand, I have three siblings and two parents whom I love dearly and who dearly love me. I still have amazing friends. My dog still looks at me with an incomprehensible level of admiration. I have an amazing job. Those extra ninety minutes didn't have any impact on the important things in my life.

This is why people need to stop getting so hung up on pace. Some people I have helped in their running lives have expressed a deep interest in running a half or a full marathon, but they hesitate because "I'm just too slow." My mother is one of those people. Mom was an avid runner growing up and managed to hold a pretty darned quick pace back then (about eight minutes per mile, if memory serves me correctly). This is why she's frustrated now that her pace has dropped quite a bit because she's gotten a few more years under her belt and has been away from running for a number of years. (Just for the record: no, Mom, I'm not calling you old.)

I have completed marathons in times that range from under three hours to almost four and a half hours, and every single race was just as gratifying and satisfying as the last one and the next one. They were satisfying in different ways, but not any more or any less. Just different.

By now, I have even stopped telling fellow runners that I've run Boston. The first time I qualified, it was practically part of how I introduced myself. "Hi, my name is Josh, I'm from Oregon, I'm a Virgo, I like long walks on the beach, and I qualified to run the Boston Marathon. It's great to meet you."

Again, what a jackass I was.

A very dear friend of mine who attended that race in Boston told me how she was bragging to her friends and family that her best friend was running in the Boston Marathon. If someone else does the bragging about you, well, it's perfectly acceptable. But in running, I have found it's best to be wary of bragging about yourself and your own accomplishments. It's better to brag about the accomplishments of other people.

It's funny how life is the same way. I used to think people would notice and be impressed only if I pumped my ego and bragged about my accomplishments. I was wrong. They'll notice something, but probably only just how big a jackass you are.

Life lesson learned: *Be humble. People will notice.*

3

Failure Is Inevitable

> You, me or nobody is gonna hit as hard as life. But it ain't about how hard you hit. It's about how hard you can get hit and keep moving forward.
>
> —Rocky Balboa, played by Sylvester Stallone, speaking to his son in *Rocky Balboa*

People love an underdog. Many actors have made careers and millions of dollars playing underdogs. Why? Why does the entire United States still tear up when they watch highlights of the 1980 Olympics in which the U.S. Olympic hockey team beat the Russian team? It was a major upset. Why was the 1993 movie *Rudy* an instant classic? Why do I get goosebumps every time I watch Rocky beat Apollo Creed in *Rocky II* and Mr. T in *Rocky III*?

It's because both Rudy and Rocky fail. They fail. And fail again. And fail yet again. Just when you think they're about to succeed, they fail again. And just when you assume they're going to throw in the towel and give up, instead of giving up, they get back up. And they ultimately succeed. Many underdog Hollywood stories that inspire all of us follow that same general storyline.

The reason people seem to be obsessed with people and stories about people who fail is because people fail. Every day. I'm sure my friends and loved ones get tired of hearing me saying this, but when I wake up every morning there are only two things that are inevitable and unavoidable:

1) I'm going to make choices today
2) I'm going to fail today

Do I have to get out of bed? Nope. That's a choice. Do I have to go to work? Certainly not. But I choose to work. Do I have to tell my wife good morning and that I love her every morning? No, I don't. There's an old adage that the only two inevitable things in life are death and taxes. But paying taxes is actually another choice. You don't technically have to pay taxes. It is a choice…a choice with consequences. Just ask Al Capone about tax evasion, who could have been imprisoned for any one of countless horrific acts he was a part of, but instead could only be officially found guilty of tax evasion.

So we watch people like Daniel E. "Rudy" Ruettiger in the 1993 movie. He's an undersized, below-average student blessed with very few genetic advantages, and by sheer grit and determination, and through failure, he somehow succeeds. We watch him struggle to succeed on the big screen. *Rudy* gives us hope. It gives us inspiration. Then we can say to ourselves, "If he can do that then there is certainly hope for me." Going into detail about Rudy the movie here would take too long, but those of you who have seen it know exactly what I'm referring to. For those that haven't, I highly recommend seeing it. Don't forget your Kleenex.

As runners, we are not strangers to failure. One of the things I constantly tell people I coach is that while they're training for and running a marathon, there is so much that can go wrong. And so little that can go right. The hard thing to remember while going through failure is that it's the failures that actually make us stronger.

If I listed all of my running failures, they would create a book rivaling *War and Peace* in length, so I'm not going there. But there are some of my more spectacular failures I want to share. First, I'd like to point out that I use the term "failure" pretty loosely in some of these situations. If I'm coaching a runner and she sets her eyes on a 3:40 time as a goal and runs a 3:42, I don't necessarily consider that a failure. She succeeded in a lot of ways just through the process of training and running. For the sake of this chapter, however, I'm saying "failure." Here goes:

In 2009, I planned my very first full marathon in Miami with my sister Laurie. After my sixteen-mile training run, the outside of my left knee started hurting. The pain wouldn't go away. I had to drop out of the race. (An MRI revealed an inflamed IT band.)

In 2011, my training was humming along like it never had before, and I had an aggressive goal of running a sub-2:50 time. All of my training runs were pointing toward that being more than realistic. Running the relatively flat Oklahoma City Memorial Marathon seemed like the perfect run, but when I woke up on race day, there were thunderstorms accompanied by 30 MPH winds, pouring rain, and hail. Weather threw a wrench into my plans. While I still ran a 2:59, which stands to this day as my personal record, I still wonder what my time would have been with better conditions.

The 2012 Boston Marathon and its 87-degree weather. I've already discussed this, but just writing about it now makes me feel overheated.

Fresh off my very first Boston Marathon, I set my sights on the August 2012 Anchorage Marathon as my next Boston qualifier. While typically summer training and I don't get along, my training for Anchorage was going surprisingly well. This is a Sunday race, so a couple of fellow runners and I were planning to fly up on Friday to arrive in time for Saturday's packet pickup. (For non-runners, "packet pickup" refers to a set time before the race where each participant must come and pick up his packet, which contains race information, his bib, and his racing giveaway, which is usually a shirt, and other goodies.) Thursday night, while I was packing for the trip, I started feeling under the weather. When I woke up Friday morning, I had the full-on flu. I had to drop down to the half marathon and I still struggled to finish that. Yes—most rational people would point out that if I had the flu, I should have dropped out completely. But I'm too stubborn for that.

Fast forward twelve months later to the 2013 Anchorage Marathon. Again I had my sights set on a Boston qualifier. The training was going well. Eight weeks before the race, I ran eighteen miles and felt great. A week later, I set out on a nine-mile run. Four miles from home, I stepped to the side to avoid some low-hanging branches above the sidewalk I was running on. The grass was overgrown enough that it was hiding a gopher hole in the ground. Which I, of course, stepped right into with my right foot. My ankle rolled. I fell. It started swelling immediately. I knew it was a severe sprain. With no cell phone, my only option was to keep running on it—toward home—before it stiffened up. I hobbled the four miles back home, ran inside, and immediately put a frozen bag of peas on my already grapefruit-size ankle. The injury sidelined me from all running for about three and a half weeks, meaning another long run before the race just wasn't possible. Being stubborn (have I mentioned that?), I flew to Anchorage anyway and decided to try the marathon. Although I was holding a Boston qualifying pace through mile 20, at that point my legs just simply had nothing left. That's because I was undertrained. I was also in a lot of pain, but that's nothing new for us marathoners, so I was trying to show some mental toughness by telling my legs to keep running that fast. They refused.

Realistically, they simply couldn't. I ended up with a 3:18, falling short again of my Boston qualifying goal.

In 2015, my sister and I decided we wanted to run a race in which we would both qualify for Boston, after which we planned to run Boston together. Our qualifications for a race were pretty basic: sea level, relatively flat, Eastern time zone, high chances of low temperatures. After some research, we zeroed in on Myrtle Beach, South Carolina. Both of our trainings were going solid, and it looked like our goal was in sight. So here's what happens: We get to the starting line, our excitement at an all time high, and we're off with the gun. There's a big smile on my face as I pass the first mile marker. And suddenly my back tightens up. It's not debilitating, or even painful, really, but I can definitely feel it's super tight. Which has never happened to me before. Since it wasn't painful, I didn't think much of it and just kept on running. The issue when your back tightens up is that it affects everything else through your body. It alters your stride. Your stride being altered for five miles is manageable. Your stride being altered for 26.2 miles…that's a big problem. By mile 8, my legs were so fatigued I didn't think I could go on. I managed to hobble through the half marathon, and then I practically collapsed at the finish line, frustrated beyond belief. But I found the silver lining as I watched Laurie cross with her Boston qualifying time achieved. We celebrated!

The list of times I failed goes on and on. The point I'm making in telling these stories is that failure is inevitable for everyone. We often look at the people we idolize, whether they're athletes or musicians or CEOs, and we assume that life is easy for them. We assume they never fail. But what is the reality for those people who are the most successful? They probably fail more often than almost everyone else.

Here's the important point: They're successful because every time they fall down, they don't stay down. They get up. As Rocky said, life ain't about how hard you can hit. It's about how hard you can get hit and keep moving forward.

The more times we get pushed down, the harder it is to keep getting up. If you're trying to get into law school, the first time you're told no is easier to take than the seventh. Rudy's first rejection by Notre Dame stung a lot less than the fifth rejection. But I guarantee you that the gratification of finally succeeding makes all those failures worth it.

The easy path in situations where you fail is to just give up. Giving up is safe because you know you're not going to get pushed down again. That's when you ask yourself, "Why would I put myself through all that heartache again?" The reality is most people don't give it another try. They don't set themselves up to be pushed down again. Most of us choose not to put ourselves out there. We choose not to set lofty goals. The goals we do set, we choose not to share with other people so if we don't make it, they won't laugh at us.

Why do most people choose these paths? Because they might fail again.

But I have news for you. You cannot avoid failure. It's everywhere. And, quite frankly, it's not a bad thing. It's simply part of the process.

> Just about anything worth doing is worth doing better, which means, of course, that there will be failure. That's not a problem, it's merely a step along the way.
> —Seth Godin

Think about the business world. Everyone has been laid off. Tried for a promotion and gotten looked over. Think about school. Aimed for an A and received a C.

> Show me a man who has never made a mistake, and I will show you one who has never tried anything new.
> —Anonymous

I'm not making an argument that I enjoy failure. Or that failure is fun. Or that you have to decide to like it. I don't use the word "hate" very often, but it's fitting here: I HATE FAILURE. I absolutely cannot stand to fail. When I set out to accomplish something and fall short for whatever reason, it eats at me. I lose sleep over it. I can't think of anything else all day. All night, too.

You don't have to enjoy failure. But you do have to accept its inevitability.

Running. Career. School. Friendships. Marriage and relationships. Life in general. There will be times when you fail.

As some have said, you've got to be willing to take the hits.

Life lesson learned: *Failure is inevitable. How you respond to it is up to you.*

4

It's Heart That Matters

> I've always believed that if you put in the work, the results will come. I don't do things half-heartedly. Because I know if I do, then I can expect half-hearted results.
>
> —Michael Jordan

Looking back on my days as a kid growing up in Oregon, it is now obvious to me that I had no grasp of the difference between *want* and *need*. Which is not much different from most kids. When we're young and see our favorite sports figure, actor, musician, or whoever we happen to be idolizing at that moment, we want to be exactly like them. So if they're wearing a certain article of clothing or endorsing some other product, we don't just want it. *We crave it. We need it.*

While I had a happy childhood with a great family, good hot meals, and a clean, sturdy house in a safe neighborhood, my family didn't have a whole lot of money for extras. Mom and Dad were always good about saving to make sure we four kids could participate in all of the extracurricular activities we wanted to, but with four of us, there simply wasn't enough money to go around to buy us all the top-of-the-line gear, shoes, instruments, etc.

That was frustrating to me. To this day, I don't think I have ever wanted anything as badly as I wanted a pair of Air Jordans, the shoes made famous by a gentleman who may have had more impact on his sport than anyone has ever impacted any other sport. If you were a young boy in the 1990s, you idolized Michael Jordan. It was a fact of life. It is thus no coincidence that Nike's Air Jordan shoes sold like hotcakes despite their $100+ price tag (which, at the time, was borderline absurd to pay for a pair of shoes). Jordan's popularity and the popularity of his shoes was so strong, in fact, that Nike still puts out a yearly line of Air Jordan shoes to this day, years after his retirement.

So you can imagine my dismay and disgust when Mom and I would head to the store for that year's pair of basketball shoes for me and we walked right past the Air Jordans to arrive at the X Brand aisle where the shoes cost around $20. That's what my parents could afford.

"Cool kids don't wear this crap," I always said to myself as I looked at the X Brand shoes. Then I wondered how my mother could even dare to think I would even stand a slim chance at keeping up with all of the other players while I was wearing such subpar shoes. Like P.F. Flyers made famous by generations before me, I was convinced that a fresh, sparkling pair of Jordans would make me run faster and jump higher than all the other kids at school. "Mom," I always said, but only to myself, "I would most certainly be the best player out there if you would just fork over the extra dough for these shoes."

This same battle happened every year before baseball season, when I was convinced I needed a bat of my own and a new glove. Every season, I was sure I could persuade Mom and Dad to buy me my own brand new TPX bat and a brand-new Rawlings Gold Glove Series Heart of the Hide glove.

How many times did I win that battle? A big fat goose egg. Looking back on those days, as I look back at many things I have done, I wish I could go back in time and take a different approach.

My teammates had a variety of quality of equipment. Some of them had the best, brand-new, top-of-the-line gear money could buy. They had it every year, too. (I'm still confused as to what they did with last year's "used" equipment.) Some guys had above-average equipment that might have been a year or two old. They usually bought new stuff every couple years. And then there were kids like me, who got a glove from his uncle as a Christmas present when he was thirteen. He used it all the way through high school. Or the kid who used the only bat he ever owned, which was bought used at a Play it Again Sports his freshman year of high school. (I still have the glove, which was given to me by my Uncle Jon, by the way).

My teammates also had a range of skill levels, from the guys who would dazzle you from an early age to those other guys whose coordination made you strongly question the equilibrium of their brains. I sometimes wondered if some people actually had to try to be that uncoordinated.

But here's the kicker: those two concepts—quality of equipment and level of skill—had absolutely no correlation to each other. There were amazing players, some much better than me, who stepped out onto the court or the field with hand-me-down gear that looked barely usable. And there were other guys who were wearing $1,000 worth of gear and rode the bench because, quite frankly, they sucked. Early on, I made the mistake of thinking there was a correlation between gear and skill. But there wasn't then, and there isn't now.

The same is true for running.

Even in a sport filled with grown-ups, I observe countless people making that same misjudgment. They seem to think they can run better when they're wearing expensive gear.

After I got my first few races under my belt, I received a phone call from my sister Jennie. She and I grew up super close and remain close. She and I are the closest in age and were the last two in the house after Luke and Laurie left for college. That's why, as young kids, we did everything together. So when she phoned me, I was flattered to learn she had apparently gotten some level of inspiration from my running and was interested in getting into a training program for a race of her own.

As I later learned, after she had casually mentioned her intentions to a few of her co-workers, they jumped at the opportunity to give her all the advice that, in their minds, she needed to help her along. During our conversation, however, she seemed almost depressed. While she had been excited to jump right into training, she eventually came clean as to why she was calling me.

"Josh," she confessed, "I just don't think I can afford to get into running. It's too expensive."

I was floored. *Can't afford it?* That wasn't logical. I was baffled. *Can't afford what?* At this stage of my running career, when this conversation took place, as far as equipment was concerned, I was a minimalistic runner. I had no iPod, no GPS, not one piece of Dri-FIT clothing, and I most certainly didn't have one of those goofy looking hats they make for runners. I still don't. (And I wonder…would it kill those companies to make a moisture-wicking hat with some style?).

All of Jennie's co-workers had made it sound like she absolutely had to have all of these things. Want to run your first 5k? Here is a list of what you "need": iPod, GPS watch, water belt, compression spandex shorts, Dri-FIT socks, shorts and shirts, protein shake powder, professionally fit expensive shoes, a gym membership, no-slip sunglasses, spandex pants, a water/wind-proof running jacket, Dri-FIT gloves, and a Dri-FIT stocking cap for cold weather. Price tag? Probably in the thousands of dollars. And not a single thing on this list will run the 3.1 miles for you. Or the 26.2 miles. Or whatever distance you're trying to run.

Reality check for any runner: no matter what your experience level is, you *don't need any* of that stuff. You simply *want* it. I sometimes chuckle when I see someone at the starting line of a race who looks like a running store threw up all over them.

You see it in the business world, too. A businessman casually strolls into the conference room wearing a $4,000 suit, carrying the finest briefcase money can buy, and equipped with all the latest tech gear from Apple, plus a high-dollar Bluetooth in his ear. Does that mean that guy is any more or less effective in sales or at running a company than anyone else? Is he the best at whatever job he has? Of course not. He just happened to have spent a lot of money on his wardrobe.

Jennie had a non-running experience that drove this lesson home. In her own words:

I learned to never judge a book by its cover. At Best Buy, a very well dressed, clean cut man plowed into me, knocking me into a DVD rack, which thankfully held me up. But my armful of purchases and the DVDs all went flying while I was wobbling and trying to stay upright. Not so much as a "pardon me" was uttered. He kept going. However, a tattooed young man with a green mohawk raced over from the next aisle, helped me right myself, gathered up my purchases, and offered to walk me to the checkout stand.

Here is the kicker: Jennie was eight months pregnant when this happened. I tell this story not to encourage people to go get tattoos all over their arms and grow green mohawks, but to suggest that we all be careful when judging people—runners or non-runners or anyone else—by what they look like. Fancy, expensive gear doesn't mean anything about how strong a runner you are. Just like a mohawk doesn't mean you're weird and inconsiderate.

Now I should clarify that I always encourage any runner to acquire any piece of gear that they perceive will help them run more often, train harder, and achieve their goals. Even if it's the placebo effect working on you, if you're convinced that wearing a tie-dyed miniskirt on warm days helps your circulation and helps get your butt off the coach to get out for a run, then more power to you. I'll buy you your first one.

But my plea to the folks who are just getting into running, or who are considering it and looking for advice, is don't buy into the equipment fallacy like kids do and like I did when I was a kid. *What you want and what you need are two very different things.*

One of the reasons that running is so appealing to me, and to many other runners, is its simplicity. You go running. That's it.

So a list of what you actually need is pretty simple: shoes, socks, something to cover your genitals so as not to be arrested for public indecency, and a strip of road to run on that won't cause you to become plastered bug guts on the windshield of somebody's SUV. That's it. Shoes, shorts, and a road. Running has nothing to do with the gear.

You can't judge someone's abilities by their fancy, expensive running clothes, their ambitious training plans, and their expensive professional trainers. We judge runners by how much gusto they train with. Stores can sell you fancy clothes, suits, Bluetooths, and water belts, but no store in the world can sell you heart. Which trumps all.

The reason I've run the races I have, or why I absolutely rocked that presentation last week, isn't because of my expensive shoes or because I use a new laser pointer with all the flashy gadgets on it. I ran the races successfully because I woke up at 4 a.m. to run fifteen sets of hill intervals and do forty-five minutes of grueling core exercises while you were still sound asleep. I rocked my last presentation because I was practicing in front of a mirror for hours.

Michael Jordan was successful because of his preparation, but, like most kids, I idolized him for the wrong reasons. I thought he was born to be the greatest basketball player of all time. I was sure that if I wore the same clothes and shoes as he did, then maybe I could play remotely as well as he did.

Some of you may recall the 1997 NBA finals game when Jordan had the flu but still played. He was so sick that not only did they have to administer an IV to him at halftime, but his teammates also had to physically hold him up in the huddle during timeouts to prevent him from collapsing. They had to carry him off the floor after the game because he was so exhausted he couldn't take another step.

Jordan scored 38 that night. The Bulls won.

What should we attribute that performance to? Air Jordans? P.F. Flyers? A fancy $300 GPS watch or a trendy $4000 suit? Of course not.

He scored 38 because he had had the guts, determination, and focus to succeed despite the adversity facing him. Michael Jordan had heart.

When you're running along and hit the proverbial wall at mile 18, none of that fancy gear is going to take the next step for you. It's not going to force you to keep running even though your legs feel like they are being punched by a white-hot Mike Tyson roundhouse.

You have to earn it with grit and determination. With heart.

Sometimes we see heart in different situations, but I'll never forget a display of heart I once saw on a run. A few years back, I took my dad to the greatest museum I have ever been to: the Baseball Hall of Fame in Cooperstown, New York. We both flew into Albany on separate flights, and I arrived about three hours before he did. Knowing I would have three hours to kill, I had done some research and found a trail alongside the Hudson River. It looked perfect for running, so when I arrived and picked up my rental car, I drove to that trail, found a place to park and a restroom to change in, and started on a run.

It was a great trail and a beautiful day for a run. I was soaking in all the sights when I turned a corner, looked ahead, and saw her. I'll never forget the look on her face. Her glare branded a welt in my brain in whatever section of your brain controls fear.

It was a mother goose. She was standing smack in the middle of the trail about fifteen yards ahead. She was staring right at me. I stopped cold. If I wanted to use this section of trail, I was going to have to go through Mother Goose. And I was going to have a fight on my hands. For some folks, it may have taken some deliberation to decide what to do, but for me, it was a no-brainer. I had tangled with geese when I was a kid and had come out on the wrong end of the dispute every single time. I have been uncertain about a lot of things in my time, but on that day and on that trail, I was one hundred percent certain that I wanted nothing to do with that goose. I looked at her and she just stared right back at me with her deep, dark, beady eyes as if to say, "Come on, big boy...I DARE you!"

No stretch of trail in the history of running trails is worth messing with a Momma Goose.

I took a detour. I ran off the path and made sure not to get anywhere near her. As I kept an eye on her, I could see her still staring at me following me the entire way and probably hoping I would slip up ever so slightly and give her the window of opportunity she needed to get a taste of the meaty flesh on my legs.

I am a grown man weighing in at 245 pounds. That goose couldn't have weighed more than twenty pounds. Yet she showed no fear of me, whereas I was practically searching for a new pair of underwear. Fact of life: any time something that weighs twenty pounds shows no fear facing a fight with something that weighs 245 pounds, put your money on the twenty-pounder every time. That goose would have torn me apart because in her mind she was fighting for her own or her offspring's lives. Her guts and determination. Her heart. That's what she had, what I didn't.

We also sometimes see displays of heart in people we know, love, and admire. And it makes us admire them even more. I can remember when I was ten years old and my sister Jennie was a freshman in high school. Softball season had just started, and she was practicing with the varsity team because her reputation as a pretty darned good catcher had preceded her. The coaches were evaluating her to see if she could start as a freshman on the varsity team. Dad and I went to pick her up from practice since she was too young to have a driver's license. We arrived toward the end of practice, while the team was doing laps around the field. For a minute, it looked like Jennie was bringing up the rear. She was way behind everyone else.

"Dad," I said, "why is Jennie so far behind everyone?"
"She's not," he responded. "She's about to lap everyone else."
"Well, how come she's so much faster than everyone else?"
"She's not faster," he said. "She's just tougher."

Looking back on that day, I realize that Dad wasn't trying to say she was actually tougher than anyone else on that softball field. What he meant was that she was just working twice as hard as everyone else. How else could, or should, a freshman be outperforming everyone else?

Jennie went on to be a four-year starter at the most difficult position on a baseball or softball field, a catcher, for one of the top softball teams in the state. She was twice voted to the all-state team and was once named first team all-state, indicating that the coaches and the media had voted her as the best catcher in the state. She went on to play at the Division 1 level.

As someone who attended almost all of her high school and summer league games, I can tell you without a doubt that she was the envy of every single opposing coach and every opposing pitcher. Not because of her prowess as a batter, because very few elite, defensive catchers are good hitters, and she was no exception. It was her intelligence about the game and the way she approached it which set her apart. She put her teammates first at all times, always had their backs (especially her pitcher's), and nobody ever questioned which player out of the eighteen on the field was playing the hardest. She had more impact on the game than any player in any given game because of how she approached her teammates, her coaches, and the game in general.

Every aspect of life works the same way. I have never heard a true success story tell his or her story without attributing their success to hard work. No matter what aspect of life you're trying to succeed at, the one true constant in the success equation is hard work. Grit. Determination. Heart.

Want to be a better parent? Spend more time with your kids and concentrate on being a better parent. Trying to climb the ladder at your accounting firm? Stop goofing off at the water cooler or on Facebook during half the day. Jealous of how much more successful someone else's marriage is? It isn't because they're lucky. I guarantee you they have to work hard every single day at having a good marriage.

Running is the same. When you see someone cross the finish line at a marathon, it's not because they were blessed with the genetic gift to be able to run 26.2 miles. Or even one mile. It's not because they spent thousands of dollars on the gear everyone else told them they *needed*. It's because they worked for it. Do you want to try and run a half marathon but you can't currently even make it a quarter mile? No problem. Run an eighth of a mile. Next week run a quarter. The week after that, run half a mile. Keep working at it. Pour your heart into a sensible training plan. You'll get there eventually.

Life lesson learned: *The gear doesn't make the runner. Or the business person. Or the parent. Or the spouse.*

It's heart that matters

5

Be Patient

> It's not the will to win that matters. Everyone has that. It's the will to prepare to win that matters.
> —Bear Bryant

One of the trendiest topics out in today's business world that we like to discuss, analyze, train, and operate on is the personality profile. Identifying, analyzing, and managing around someone's personality type certainly isn't new, but it has become a focal point of almost any business management training. We find baby boomers learning to work with Generation Y'ers. Introverts being productive around extroverts. People who crave change versus those who cringe and run away from it.

Whether you use the DiSC Personality Test, the Myers Briggs Type Indicator, or any of the other personality tests that are available today, you soon learn that they all speak to the same personality types and tendencies. Each personality profile system will help spell out how personalities and styles differ, and one of the differences you find in those different personalities are the pace and speed at which those people live their lives.

Some folks—I like to call them the Wall Street traders—are constantly on the move, with fast talking and fast walking. They don't take time to mull over details. They always seem to be in a hurry.

Other people—let's call them three toed sloths—move at the proverbial snail's pace and go so slow sometimes it makes the Wall Streeters' heads explode. There is no sense of urgency with them, as opposed to those who seem to live their life by a sense of urgency.

When it comes to health, fitness, and weight loss, most people tend to want to be like the fast-moving Wall Street traders. They want to lose weight and get in shape in a month, and if they think their progress is too slow, they give up quickly and move on to something else. Consistent diet and exercise aren't complicated. Good health is not rocket science, and success in weight loss, diet, and exercise doesn't require any kind of complex formula to work. But they do take time and dedication.

A friend recently called me and asked for some advice and help on getting in shape. She told me she had a trip to Florida planned, but she hadn't exercised in quite some time. Now she wanted some coaching on how to get back in shape and toned up for those days when she'd be lying on the beach in a swimsuit. In other words, swimsuit season was approaching and she was looking to firm up.

I'm always more than happy to help anyone who asks me for help getting into shape, so my first question to her was to ask how much time we had to work with before her trip. When was she leaving for Florida?

"Next week," she said.

"Next week?" I repeated. "As in *next week*? Like, seven days from today?"

"Yes. Can you help me?"

I was flabbergasted. "No," I said, "I'm sorry, but I can't help you. No trainer in the world can get any body into shape in a week. Had you called me three months ago, then I could have helped you with a few things. But there is little I can do for you in a matter of seven days."

People trying to lose weight often have the same mentality—instant weight loss—which ultimately leads to the same result. Failure. People need to remember that trying to lose that extra twenty-five pounds of jiggle from your butt, legs, and stomach is going to take some time and some work. You didn't gain that extra twenty-five pounds in a week, and you surely aren't going to lose it in a week. I should take the opportunity right here to point out that any gimmick you hear about guaranteeing significant weight loss in insignificant amounts of time is exactly that: a gimmick. Instead of listing all of the specific programs you hear about on TV, my best advice is to be wary of any promotion advertising anything that is not focused on a consistent and long-term commitment to proper nutrition and/or exercise.

Wanting everything *right now* tends to be the American way today, as the immediacy of text messaging, social media, and online shopping give us an expectation that we should be able to get answers and results right now.

But fitness and running don't work that way.

The most heartbreaking moments in my running career have come because of injuries. Everyone has minor injuries—sore feet, lost toenails, blisters, and other relatively minor inconveniences that we runners just have to learn to live with. What I'm talking about are the major injuries that knock you out of training for significant time.

I have had three different significant injuries for a total of four time-outs. IT Band problems in my left knee. Two different bouts with plantar fasciitis, once in each foot. Acute tendonitis in my left ankle. The IT Band injury caused me to have to cancel my first-ever planned full marathon, which I was supposed to run with my sister. I was devastated when I had to drop out.

Runners will tell you that running becomes an addiction, so much so that if you have to abstain from running for weeks, not to mention months, it takes a toll on your mental health. You start going nuts because you don't have that element of your life to lean on anymore. Injuries are brutal and difficult to cope with, both physically and psychologically, and that brutality tends to happen when a runner does one of two things: (1) he tries to increase his weekly mileage too quickly, or (2) she tries to come back from a major race too soon.

To clarify, sometimes a runner will perceive that their body feels great after a major run or a major race. But there are underlying issues they may not be aware of. Rather than allowing their bodies to have the proper amount of time to rest, some runners will get a bit too ambitious and get right back to running and training. And an injury results.

For all of the non-runners reading this, I should point out that injuries in different sports often occur in different ways. Generally speaking, most injuries in the major American sports like football and basketball happen in an instant: a torn ACL, a broken finger. But for the most part, running injuries don't work like that.

Imagine lightly dragging your fingernail across a patch of skin on your opposing arm. Do that once, and you would barely feel it. Do it ten times, and you'll still barely feel it. A hundred times, and it will start to get annoying. And by the time you get to ten thousand of these "light" scratches, you may not have an arm left. That's how running injuries occur. We don't get our arm broken because a 260-pound linebacker crashed into it. We develop stress fractures in our feet and inflamed tendons in our hips after hundreds of miles on the asphalt. So we need to learn to give those parts of our bodies time to heal and recover before we get back to "scratching" them.

In other words, our American attitude of wanting results right now makes us try to do too much too fast when we shouldn't make such strenuous efforts. Not all, but many, injuries would go away if we could just slow down a little bit. But that's one of life's tough qualities we have to master.

Patience.

Runners have to absolutely learn patience. Because if we don't, the likely result is injury. If you're impatient, your likelihood of disaster is fairly high.

Patience is one of those lessons that ends up making runners crazy because one certainty in training for a race is that things aren't going to go as planned. That typically means training goes slower than we had hoped. You're going to get the flu. Or a sore heel. Or your legs will feel like jello for an entire week. Maybe your life suddenly gets hectic and you end up having to push back your weekly long run. All of which mean your training is going to slow down.

But slowing down is especially frustrating for runners because we runners tend to be eternally optimistic. When we create a training plan detailing each and every activity specific for each day, we get excited and assume that this time it's going to be different. We're going to follow this plan the entire way without any hiccups and get that elusive personal record we've been trying for.

But, as I said before, things never go as planned. Hardly anything ever does, and especially in running. One of the reasons marathon runners put their running accomplishments on their resumes is because that shows recruiters and hiring managers that they can roll with the punches, fight through adversity, and still finish what they set out to do months or even years ago.

There is no room for impatience. If your next long run is scheduled to be fifteen miles, but you decide you're ready for more and run twenty, you're going to regret it. Your body isn't ready to run that much distance, and injury is the most likely result from that decision. You may feel okay after the twenty-mile run. Even good the next day. But it'll eventually come back to bite you. As in running, many baseball careers seem to have been ruined because someone in the head office decided to rush the team's prospect into the big leagues before they're ready. After the new guy has been eaten up by big league pitching or hitting, his psyche is forever crushed.

Many of our race plans have been blown to pieces because people mistakenly take the approach, "To heck with only running ten. I feel GREAT! Let's run twice that!" And a week later, they wonder where this stress fracture came from. Their training seemed to be going so well, so why did this stress fracture suddenly appear?

Because you were impatient. That's why.

After a race, we can sit around and become stir crazy thinking that rather than resting, we should be back out on the asphalt where we're sure we belong. Running. In reality, we should be off the asphalt. Resting.

What we really need is just a small dose of patience.

I read a lot of books, and three of my favorites touch on the subject of being patient in order to be successful: *Outliers* by Malcolm Gladwell, *Talent Is Overrated* by Geoff Colvin, and *The Talent Code* by Daniel Coyle. In all three of these books, the authors assert that in order to display a mastery of something, it takes a minimum of 10,000 hours of practice. One author argues that while it takes that many hours to master something, it takes twice that—20,000 hours—to master it to the point of being able to teach it.

To put that into perspective, let's say you're learning to play the violin and you want to master the art of playing. To reach that goal, you would have to consistently practice four hours a day, five days a week for over almost ten years. After that decade of repetitive practice, you'll be able to stand in front of a crowd and masterfully deliver a piece of music that brings the audience to their feet. Most of your audience might comment that delivering that piece of music so masterfully must have been incredibly difficult. They would be wrong. Playing that music wasn't hard in itself. What was hard was that decade of consistent, intentional practice. Once you've done the practicing, the delivery is easy by comparison.

You'll read this elsewhere in this book: running a marathon isn't hard compared to training to run a marathon. It's related to the Bear Bryant quote at the beginning of this chapter. Because a lot of people I have known want to run a marathon, but only a small percentage of them actually want to put in the work required to run a marathon. Bear Bryant is right on.

Here's a paraphrase of Bryant's quote in my own words: *Executing isn't difficult. Preparing to execute well is.*

Delivering a breathtaking keynote speech takes thirty minutes. Learning to be a top-notch public speaker takes a lifetime. A concert lasts an hour or two, but mastering your instrument takes decades.

It's no secret to anyone who knows me that I'm a big fan of the band Metallica. Whether you like their music or not, you should know that very few other bands can rival their success and that their success can be attributed to decades of dedication and hard work. I once read a story about the band preparing for its thirtieth anniversary by playing for four consecutive nights at the world-famous Fillmore in San Francisco. The story told how the band was doing four-hour sound checks and eight-hour rehearsals every day for a week to prepare for the shows. This band, which has been putting out bestselling records and playing to sold-out venues for decades, was still putting in ten-to-twelve-hour days to prepare for four shows.

Preparing to execute is difficult.

And it takes patience.

Most of us don't want to put in the time to prepare for something (a marathon, a game, a performance) because we simply don't have the patience. But patience is what is the key to success in anything. Those who lack patience have a difficult time mastering any craft.

This also holds true for interacting with people. We have all had our spats with friends, co-workers, and family members. Often, these conflicts are a result of our losing patience with that person. I used to work with college students and have supervised a handful of employees who were right out of college. Sometimes those students and fresh graduates did things and conducted business in a way which defied logic and made my brain hurt. I constantly had to remind myself that I have significantly more experience than they do. I also have to tell myself that I made many of the same mistakes when I was in their shoes.

Sometimes I missed a deadline. Or forgot to respond to an email. Or screwed up a report. Or did something else stupid. I've had to tell myself I've made just as many mistakes as the next person. Maybe more. But rather than continuing to dwell on things that annoy me, now I try my best to focus on the good things those people do.

Having patience with people's imperfections is one of the most valuable qualities anyone who manages a team can possess. It is also, not coincidentally, one of the toughest to master. I'm still certainly a novice at it. I catch myself feeling impatient every single day. I'm sure it's something we all struggle with every day.

As I write this, I think about that quality of patience and relate it to injuries I've had in running. I also think about the skills I constantly have to work to improve.

Being patient and staying committed and consistent are key.

Ten thousand hours is a lot of practice. And that's the hard part because preparing to execute well is difficult. It takes patience, enormous amounts of patience.

Life lesson learned: *Be Patient.*

6

Running Is Cheaper than Therapy

A very common reason, maybe the most common reason, people give for not working out and exercising is that their schedule is so full with work, family, volunteering, and other activities, that they simply don't have the time to fit exercising into their days. Exercise is lower on their priority list than almost anything else, so it almost always takes a back seat. I understand that. If you truly only have ninety "extra" minutes in a given day and you have to choose between dedicating that time to your family or dedicating it to exercise, you should choose family. One hundred times out of one hundred.

But I see running as a time-saver in my life. It's an investment. I recall a business trip I went on in the Northeast awhile back. It was unbelievably exhausting. I was emotionally and psychologically drained while facilitating a discussion and a negotiation from Thursday through Saturday.

When I flew back home on Sunday morning, still emotionally drained, I could only think of one thing. *I needed a run.* Bad. I felt like a crack fiend who needed his fix. So I went straight home, changed clothes, and drove a few miles to a local lake and immediately started running around the lake. Thanks to the music on my iPod, the sunshine, the lake itself and everything else in my surroundings, I was completely lost in the moment…until I returned to reality ten miles later. It was amazing how much better I felt then.

My point is that while I understand people putting many things as higher priorities than running, I have a tough time wrapping my head around the claim that some people make that they just don't have enough time to work out.

I hold the opposite claim to be true. I don't have enough time *to not work out*.

I am much more emotionally healthy and more productive when I do daily vigorous exercise. I sleep better. I have more energy all day. I'm in a better mood and seek out productive activities. Investing ninety minutes in exercise in the morning makes me more productive for the rest of the day.

We all need some sort of emotional/mental/physical outlet that we can turn to when we're having a difficult time. For some, it may be intellectual in nature, like a new book to read. Others, however, may turn to an unhealthy habit like substance abuse or over-eating. For me, it's physical exertion. That's the outlet which suits me best.

My high school and college days are where that outlet was born, although at the time I didn't realize what was happening. My parents went through their divorce during my senior year of high school, and while those sorts of things are never easy, this one was pretty brutal for me and my siblings. Having to give yourself a pep talk at the age of seventeen every time you're about to see one of your parents starts to wear you down. And while I never really connected the dots back then, now I see how much physical exercise helped me survive. I was going to the gym five to six times a week during that time and doing a combination of weight training and running on the treadmill (one or two miles back then). I was in phenomenal shape.

But that's not why I went to the gym. During that time of my life the gym was one of the few constant, reliable things I had. It was something I could control. It was something I could look forward to, a place where I knew nobody would stroll up and ask me how I was doing or how my parents were holding up. Sure, I was concerned about my parents and how they were coping, but I had my own issues, too. The gym was a healthy outlet. I had to just get away from difficult issues.

That outlet continued in college. I was a fairly consistent exerciser, and I also played basketball, lifted weights, and ran on my non-basketball days, but I never really understood how valuable of an outlet that exercise was for me until March of 2004.

The Monday of spring break in 2004 found me still on campus. My plan was to hop in a car and go on a road trip to Bozeman, Montana, with some buddies to go see another buddy. We were going to spend the whole week there. As I was loading up, I heard a familiar voice yelling something at me. I turned around to see my good friend Matt parked in his pickup.

Matt, or "Sodi" to those who knew him best, lived in the fraternity house next door to my fraternity house. He and I had grown quite close over the years. We went out on the town together, went shooting together, and since we held similar leadership roles in our fraternities, did a lot of really great work together. I had come to admire his big heart, his carefree attitude, and his loud cackle of a laugh. So when I heard the voice followed by the loud cackle, I had a pretty good idea who it was.

I walked over to chat with him and find out what his plans were for spring break. I knew Sodi had just graduated, but I hadn't heard what his plans were. When I asked, he dodged the question, so I told him I was headed out of town but would call him on Saturday when I got back. We made plans to grab a beer, then I shook his hand, and we left it at that.

Fate decided to be cruel that day. I was the last person to ever speak to Sodi. Not long after our chat, he parked his pickup on a logging road just outside of town and turned his shotgun on himself.

The emotional sting of something like this is indescribable. I wouldn't wish it on anyone. People aren't born prepared to deal with a friend's suicide or anything else like that, and there is no manual that I know of that will guide you through it. When I heard what had happened to my friend, I started searching for a way to cope with the sadness.

As a guy who grew up never having had any in-depth discussions about how you feel and what emotions you're dealing with, I was stuck trying to find some way to cope with Sodi's death. Some way, other than talking it out, to deal with the emotional hurt I was in. And I was in a world of hurt.

At first, I tried to ignore it. In fact, the day I found out about Sodi's death, I was hanging out with a group of friends. It was hours before I was able to break the news to them. They were beside themselves that I hadn't mentioned it earlier. The next thing I tried was to gather all my friends—Sodi's friends—at our favorite campus watering hole and drink our emotions away.

Now, I'm not a medical doctor, and I've never even taken a single class in psychology. But my plea to everyone reading this book is *don't ever use alcohol as an emotional coping mechanism.* I tried it, and my emotional and mental pain got five times worse. It turned me into a wreck, and I had nothing to show for it except for an expensive bar tab and a nasty hangover.

The only thing I could think of to do next was to go for a run. I felt horrible, both emotionally and physically, and I figured that getting outside for a quick three-mile run would at least help me sweat out the toxins from the night before and physically help me feel better. So that's what I did.

So I went out to run, and, by god, not only did I physically feel better, but I felt emotionally refreshed, too. I was still crushed, but felt just a little bit better. So the next day I laced up my running shoes and did it again. And again the next day. Every day, I felt just a little bit better.

For months, even years, I was still torn up on the inside. Your mind races a mile a minute with questions and with blame—blaming yourself, blaming your friend (I was still blaming Sodi), blaming everyone else in the world. You ask yourself a lot of "why?" questions and you agonize over wishing you could turn back the clock to make yourself see something wrong with your friend, something that was apparently there, but you were too stupid or too preoccupied to notice. You build up strong feelings of guilt. Those questions and feelings stayed with me. Even now, as I write this many years later, I feel a bit choked up.

But while all those guilt-inducing questions kept lingering in my mind, I kept running. I never missed a run. I don't think I even told anybody at the time what I was doing to cope. I just quietly got my shoes on and slipped out the door for a run to the campus dairy's covered bridge and back. It was a scenic, remote area that helped me escape from my guilt and blame.

At a time when it didn't seem like there was anything that would help me feel better, when it felt like the hurt would never go away, running was my rock. More than any other time in my life, that was when I needed that rock. I needed to be running.

I think about Sodi a lot these days. In fact, I think about him during almost every run I go on. I no longer feel the anger or confusion and I have quit second-guessing myself and asking myself how I could have handled the situation differently. I have learned from living my life and through running that dwelling on guilty thoughts isn't healthy because I can't change what he did or what I didn't do. There was nothing I could have done to stop what happened.

What I can do is remember the good times I had with him and how lucky I was to have him in my life, even though it was for a shorter time than I would have liked. I am at peace now with what happened, and on every run I smile, knowing he is somewhere up there watching over me. I could not have arrived at this acceptance without running, and in trying to turn a negative situation into a positive one, I can be glad that through all my grief and guilt I was able to discover a healthy outlet to help myself cope with difficult situations in the future.

Life lesson learned: we all need our emotional outlet, *and running is cheaper than therapy.*

7

Differences vs. Faults

It's amazing to me how much variation exists among runners. From clothing to training plans, to long-run food choices, to Gatorade versus Pediasure, we all have our own ways of going about running. It's variation, like most things in life, that keeps things interesting.

But of all things in running, the category in which nearly all of us differ is music. Music is a highly controversial topic because there are multiple levels of variation and/or disagreement. It starts with a simple yes or no question. *Should you run to music?* The old school (the traditionalists) tend to answer with a resounding NO. Some say you should simply listen to, and soak in, your surroundings. They add that there's no reason for you to distract your senses with anything else, like music. Others recommend that you should leave yourself to your thoughts and give yourself a distraction-free time slot while you run every day to reflect on the things happening in your life.

And some cite safety reasons. When Queen is belting out "Fat Bottomed Girls" in your earphones, you're less likely to hear that wandering car with a text-messaging driver possibly aimed at you. Or, if you're female, you're not likely to sense that neighborhood creep trying to sneak up behind you.

Those reasons are valid and have sound logic. I can see those points of view.

But I choose to take a different approach. While I understand what the traditionalists are saying, I take the musical approach. I love to listen as I run. In fact, I never run intentionally without music, except if I'm running with someone else or unless my iPod is dead or I don't have it with me. I run with music. Always.

While I agree that when I run I love to get lost in my thoughts and forget about anything and everything going on around me, I find I can do the thinking more easily with music channeling through my brain.

Music is a great motivator for me when I'm running. If I'm struggling and need a pick-me-up, sometimes just the right song will come on the iPod and it helps me keep pushing. It's also extremely helpful for me during a race. I even go as far as strategically crafting a playlist and intentionally putting motivating songs on right when I know I'll need them (usually at miles 16 to 20, for the proverbial "wall").

Although many races have earphones on the forbidden list, I have yet to find a race outside of the triathlon world that actually enforces that ban. I'm not sure if they actually want earphones forbidden or if they list them simply for liability reasons.

But that particular argument will probably last forever, and the traditionalists will go on shaking their heads at us iPod bearers.

There is even more disagreement, however, among those of us who don headphones on each and every run: we argue about what music we prefer to listen to. It's a tough question to answer because there is a difference between the music I like listening to and music I like running to. For example, I love country music. Especially George Strait. I listen to country music all of the time. But how many George Strait songs or country songs in general, do I have on my running playlists? Maybe three. Country music is great music, but it's horrible to work out to. Listening to a song about David Allan Coe's mother getting "run over by a damned old train" may be fun on a Friday night, but it doesn't really help pump me up.

On the flip side, even though Eminem has some of the best music to pump you up during a workout, you'll rarely catch me playing his music just to listen to for fun on a Saturday afternoon.

So even when friends and family have asked what music I run to, I have always been hesitant to share my running playlist. To start, if any of my buddies were to get their hands on my running playlist, several of the songs on it would probably make them burst out into loud, hysterical laughter, after which they'd demand I forfeit my "man card" to them.

There are as many different types of running playlists as there are runners. So if I post mine, it simply shows what I like to listen to, which will be, at minimum, slightly different from anyone else's playlist. And because playlists are also always evolving, my favorite workout music today is much different from what I listened to twelve months ago. In fact, by the time you're reading this, my list below is sure to be out of date.

Lastly, no matter what songs I put up as my favorites, there will be folks who are critical about specific songs. They ask, how could I dare leave their favorites off my list. Yes, posting a list of my favorite running songs is bound to bring on some controversy, but I have finally just decided to say the heck with it and write about it. Controversy be dammed! (See the appendix to this chapter for my complete playlist.)

So let the controversy begin now. This is one of those fun debates in which any group engages. Not just runners. What kind of music should you listen to while you're running? From Justin Bieber fans to metalheads to folks who are so apathetic about music they think that Johnny Cash is some cockamamie government bailout program, there is a huge variety of music. But that's a good thing! As they say, variety is a spice of life.

There are certain genres, bands, and even individual songs that I have never and probably will never understand. And why anyone would ever choose to listen to that stuff is beyond my capability to understand. I just don't understand some of the songs some people choose to include on their running and/or workout playlists. Of course, they'll say the same thing about the music I listen to and choose to run to. I'm sure there's a large group of people who would be befuddled by the music I listen to.

Neither choice is wrong. We're just different.

A friend of mine recently took up running as a means of coping with emotional stress during a nasty divorce. He was having a tough time figuring out how to manage his life, and one day he just decided to go for a run. Several marathons later, he's hooked.

I couldn't be happier for my friend, as he has found a healthy outlet to use as a coping mechanism. Good for him. It has become painfully obvious, however, that we have differences of opinion when it comes to training and running. He swears by group training. Running with other folks. I prefer flying solo. When he first decided to get serious about training, he decided he needed some help and support, so he joined a local running group. He still does group training to this day.

My friend and I discovered our difference of opinion during a baseball game. Our conversation was actually pretty comical, as it reminded me a lot of a tennis match. Two people with opposite viewpoints volleying opinions back and forth. One who detests running with other people, and the other who wouldn't have it any other way. To be sure, our conversation was not adversarial and it didn't get heated, but we were both clearly quite firm in our opinions. After about ten minutes of this verbal tennis match, both of us trying to sell the other on why our way was the way to go, we agreed on the important part: we had both found training methods that worked well for us. And ultimately, that's the most important point. Neither of us is right or wrong. We just have different needs and different philosophies.

He enjoys the camaraderie of group training, not only while running but for socializing afterwards, when you go grab a beer and some food after a good hard run. He likes the accountability the group gives you to make sure you go out and run even when you don't feel like it. He likes the coaches involved in his group who monitor the runners during runs and counsel them through whatever hardships they might be facing. He likes it when other people bounce ideas and stories off each other.

All valid, valuable points.

As social as a person as I tend to be, running is the only thing I have found that I truly prefer doing alone. I enjoy the solitary aspects of running. I like it that I'm on my own schedule and not restricted by the schedule of a group. I'm also at a point in my running career that I don't need the accountability anymore. I'm a self-starter. I get out and run, and (if anything) sometimes I run too much. I like that fact that since I'm always "on" whenever I'm traveling for work, which is constantly, and I'm hardly ever by myself, sometimes not until very late at night, running has become my solitary outlet. My time to recharge solo. I like knowing that no matter what happens tomorrow, when I'm running, I'm free from phone calls, emails, text messages, discussions, and other kinds of stress. When I'm out running alone, I don't have to answer to anyone but myself and the road. Which is amazingly refreshing.

Again, all valid, valuable points.

A good friend from college is now in medical school, and our philosophies on exercise have completely flip-flopped. During our days at Oregon State, she ran quite a bit for exercise. She truly enjoyed running. I, on the other hand, despised it. Yes, I would run from time to time, but I much preferred to get my exercise playing basketball. It was social, it was exciting, it was competitive, and it was familiar. I could never understand why she ran as much as she did.

But now that she's in med school, her reasons for exercise and needs in her forms of exercise are different. And now that I have the job I have, my needs have also changed. She now plays soccer. I run.

When you're going through medical school, you spend probably fourteen to sixteen hours a day either in class or with your nose in a book. I imagine the monotony and the boredom have to be maddening. She chooses soccer as her exercise because it provides a human connection and an outlet she doesn't really get with running. In other words, her exercise is a social event in med school, which is anything but social. So where her needs in exercise include human interaction, mine do not. Solo running and training appeal to me, where solitude is the last thing she's interested in.

Not right or wrong. Different viewpoints.

When it comes to people's differing opinions on running, though, the one that takes the cake is between my father and me. I'll never forget what he said to me when I was training hard to run one of my races.

"I am very proud of you and your accomplishments," he said, "and I'll be there to cheer you on. But, man, you're crazy."

Dad has become somewhat hobbled at age sixty-nine, and it's tough for him to get around. He has a broken-down body to the point that just getting out of his recliner can be difficult, so he just can't relate to someone who sometimes spends his Friday nights running fifteen miles in subfreezing weather for "fun." For us to try to agree on exercise and running is futile. As crazy as he thought running 26.2 miles was when he was in his prime, he thinks today's marathon runners are whacko. He has no fathomable grasp on why a person would run a marathon for fun. But that didn't stop him from hobbling up out of his chair to give me a giant, grin-filled, high five at mile 21 of the Columbus Marathon on my way to my first Boston qualifier. Or from stopping every Bostonian we met on our way home from the finish line to tell those complete strangers how his son just finished the Boston Marathon, and in 90-degree heat, no less. Dad and I don't understand each other's viewpoint on running. He respects that I have my viewpoint, and I respect that he has his.

My brother is like Dad. He hates running. Always has, probably always will. And he'll never understand why my sister Laurie and I do what we do. But guess what? He was there at the finish line in

Boston, along with the rest of my family. High fiving me with a smile. Because he respects our differing viewpoints and he loves his family.

Dale Carnegie, my favorite author, had a set of "golden rules" he tried to live by. One of his rules, from How to Win Friends and Influence People is *Try honestly to see things from the other person's point of view.*

That's great advice from a great man.

Whatever your running or exercise style is, neither is "correct" or "incorrect" or "better" or "worse." The only time it's incorrect or worse is when you choose to sit your lazy butt on the couch instead of getting yourself out the door for a run. Or a swim. Or a soccer game.

Group run vs. solo run. Treadmill in the gym vs. outside in the fresh air. Nike vs. Asics. Metallica vs. KC and the Sunshine Band. Music or no music. These are all fun debates we can have with fellow runners over a beer. And neither opinion is wrong. It's whatever works for each of you.

The only right or wrong, black or white, answer is a simple one: *Exercise or don't exercise.*

Everyone is unique in their own way, and we become stronger individuals when we recognize the differences between us and also understand that people aren't right or wrong in how they differ from us. They're just *different.* The friends I described above continue to be my friends because we all recognize our different philosophies and embrace those rather than criticizing them. And we're all in each others' corners any time any of us are in a race or a game.

Life lesson learned: *Recognize and accept people's differences as differences. Not faults.*

Appendix to Chapter 7

Here is my running playlist as it stands today:

1) 50 Cent – "21 Questions"
2) 50 Cent – "Hate It Or Love It"
3) 50 Cent – "If I Can't"
4) 50 Cent – "In Da Club"
5) 50 Cent – "Wanksta"
6) Adele – "Set Fire to the Rain"
7) Adele – "Someone Like You"
8) Alice in Chains – "Nutshell"
9) Amos Lee – "Windows Are Rolled Down"
10) Anna Nalick – "Breathe (2 AM)"
11) Archie Eversole – "We Ready"
12) AWOLNATION – "Sail"
13) Beastie Boys – "Sabotage"
14) Biz Markie – "Just a Friend"
15) The Black Crowes – "Seeing Things"
16) The Black Crowes – "She Talks to Angels"
17) The Black Eyed Peas – "Boom Boom Pow"
18) The Black Eyed Peas – "I Gotta Feeling"
19) The Black Eyed Peas – "Let's Get it Started (Spike Remix)"
20) Blink 182 – "I Miss You"
21) Blink 182 – "Stay Together For the Kids"
22) Blue October – "Hate Me"
23) Blues Traveler – "The Mountains Win Again"
24) Brothers Osborne – "Stay a Little Longer"
25) Bruno Mars – "24K Magic"
26) Busta Rhymes – "Break Ya Neck"
27) Busta Rhymes – "Put Your Hands Where My Eyes Could See"
28) Calvin Harris – "Feel So Close"
29) Candlebox – "Far Behind"
30) Candlebox – "You"
31) Candlebox – "Cover Me"
32) Casey Donahew Band – "Shine on Me"

33) The Chainsmokers & Coldplay – "Something Just Like This"
34) The Chainsmokers featuring Halsey – "Closer"
35) Chamillionaire – "Ridin'"
36) Chevelle – "The Red"
37) Chris Brown featuring Juelz Santana – "Run It!"
38) Club Nouveau – "Lean on Me"
39) Coldplay – "Yellow"
40) The Cranberries – "Dreams"
41) The Cranberries – "Linger"
42) The Cranberries – "Zombie"
43) Daft Punk – "One More Time"
44) Darude – "Sandstorm"
45) Des'ree – "You Gotta Be"
46) Dionne Farris – "I Know"
47) DJ Snake – "Turn Down For What"
48) DMX – "One More Road to Cross"
49) DMX – "Party Up (Up In Here)"
50) DMX – "What's My Name?"
51) DMX – "Ruff Ryders' Anthem"
52) DMX – "X Gon' Give it to Ya"
53) DMX – "Where the Hood At"
54) DMX – "Get it on the Floor"
55) Dr. Dre and Snoop Doggy Dogg – "The Next Episode"
56) Dr. Dre and Snoop Doggy Dogg – "Still"
57) Duncan Sheik – "Barely Breathing"
58) Eddie Vedder – "Hard Sun"
59) Eminem & Nate Dogg – "'Till I Collapse"
60) Eminem – "Like Toy Soldiers"
61) Eminem – "Just Lose It"
62) Eminem – "The Way I Am"
63) Eminem featuring Rihanna – "The Monster"
64) Eminem – "The Real Slim Shady"
65) Eminem – "Not Afraid"
66) Eminem – "25 to Life"
67) Eminem – "Lose Yourself"
68) Eminem featuring Rihanna – "Love the Way You Lie"
69) Eric Church – "Record Year"
70) Evanescence – "Bring Me to Life"

71) Eve – "Let Me Blow Ya Mind"
72) Fall Out Boy – "Centuries"
73) Fall Out Boy – "My Songs Know What You Did in the Dark"
74) Fat Joe featuring Ja-Rule & Ashanti – "What's Luv?"
75) Filter – "Take a Picture"
76) Finger Eleven – "One Thing"
77) Finger Eleven – "Paralyzer"
78) Flo Rida – "My House"
79) Floater – "Cinema"
80) Floater – "The Sad Ballad of Danny Boy"
81) Florence + the Machine – "Shake it Out"
82) Fort Minor – "Remember the Name"
83) The Game featuring 50 Cent – "How We Do"
84) Gnarls Barkley – "Crazy"
85) Godsmack – "Shine Down"
86) Hoobastank – "Crawling in the Dark"
87) Hoobastank – "Running Away"
88) Hoobastank – "The Reason"
89) Imagine Dragons – "Natural"
90) Imagine Dragons – "Whatever It Takes"
91) Imagine Dragons featuring Lil Wayne – "Believer"
92) Jackson Browne – "Running on Empty"
93) Jason Boland & the Stragglers – "Outlaw Band"
94) Jason Derulo – "Want to Want Me"
95) Jay Z & Linkin Park – "Numb/Encore"
96) Jerrodd Niemann – "Shinin' On Me"
97) Jimmy Eat World – "Hear You Me"
98) Justin Timberlake featuring Timbaland – "SexyBack"
99) Justin Timberlake – "Rock Your Body"
100) Justin Timberlake – "Drink You Away"
101) Justin Timberlake – "Can't Stop The Feeling"
102) Kanye West featuring Jamie Foxx – "Gold Digger"
103) Kenny Chesney – "Somewhere With You"
104) Leona Lewis – "Bleeding Love"
105) Linkin Park – "Breaking the Habit"
106) Linkin ParK – "Numb"
107) Linkin Park – "Shadow of the Day"
108) Ludacris – "What's Your Fantasy"

109) Lupe Fiasco – "The Show Goes On"
110) Marilyn Manson – "The Beautiful People"
111) Mark Ronson featuring Bruno Mars – "Uptown Funk"
112) Mary J. Blige – "Family Affair"
113) Mase – "Feel So Good"
114) Michael Jackson – "Jam"
115) Michael Jackson – "Wanna Be Startin' Somethin'"
116) Michael Jackson – "Scream"
117) Michael Jackson – "Don't Stop 'Til You Get Enough"
118) Michael Jackson – "Rock With You"
119) Michael Jackson – "Billie Jean"
120) Michael Jackson – "Beat It"
121) Michael Jackson – "Thriller"
122) Michael Jackson – "Bad"
123) Michael Jackson – "Smooth Criminal"
124) Michael Jackson – "The Way You Make Me Feel"
125) Michael Jackson – "Man in the Mirror"
126) Michael Jackson – "Dirty Diana"
127) Michael Jackson – "Black or White"
128) Muse – "Madness"
129) Natalie Imbruglia – "Torn"
130) Nathaniel Rateliff & The Night Sweats – "S.O.B."
131) Naughty by Nature – "Hip Hop Hooray"
132) Nelly featuring City Spud – "Ride Wit Me"
133) Nelly – "Just a Dream"
134) Nelly – "Hot in Herre"
135) Nelly – "#1"
136) Nelly Furtado – "Promiscuous"
137) New Radicals – "You Get What You Give"
138) NF – "Let You Down"
139) OneRepublic – "Apologize"
140) OneRepublic – "Counting Stars"
141) Outkast featuring Killer Mike – "The Whole World"
142) Outkast – "Hey Ya!"
143) Outkast – "Ms. Jackson"
144) Pink – "Don't Let Me Get Me"
145) Pink – "Just Like a Pill"
146) Pink – "Whatever You Want"
147) Pitbull featuring Ke$ha – "Timber"

148) Prince – "Purple Rain"
149) Puddle of Mudd – "Control"
150) Puddle of Mudd – "Blurry"
151) Radiohead – "High and Dry"
152) Randy Rogers Band – "This Time Around"
153) Reckless Kelly – "1952 Vincent Black Lightning"
154) Rihanna featuring Jay Z – "Umbrella"
155) Robin Thicke featuring T.I. & Pharrell – "Blurred Lines"
156) Saliva – "Click Click Boom"
157) Seven Mary Three – "Cumbersome"
158) Simple Plan – "Addicted"
159) Smashing Pumpkins – "Today"
160) Smashing Pumpkins – "Mayonnaise"
161) Snoop Dogg & Wiz Khalifa featuring Bruno Mars – "Young, Wild & Free"
162) Staind – "Mudshovel"
163) Thirty Seconds to Mars – "The Kill"
164) Three Days Grace – "Never Too Late"
165) Train – "Mississippi"
166) Trapt – "Headstrong"
167) Trick Daddy – "Let's Go"
168) Usher featuring Lil Jon & Ludacris – "Yeah!"
169) Wiz Khalifa – "Black and Yellow"
170) Wiz Khalifa featuring Charlie Puth – "See You Again"
171) Metallica – Just about all of them (seriously—way too many to list here)

8

Pay It Forward

No matter how old I grow to be, I'll never forget the feeling I had as a kid on Christmas Eve and Christmas morning. My excitement was a combination of seeing what Santa brought me that year and knowing that I was going to be able to spend all day with my family. Eating turkey, cranberry sauce, and pumpkin pie while spending quality time with my family was the best time of the year.

And it was for my parents, too. Christmas in our house was a huge deal because my parents made it a huge deal. To this day, in fact, Christmas is a big deal to me no matter where I am or what I'm doing. My parents made it a big deal because that's what it was to them. They liked it for a lot of the same reasons we kids did—the quality time with the family, the great food, the Christmas music, a fire going in the fireplace, and a nice, relaxing day. The biggest reason they liked Christmas so much was that they loved seeing the faces of their kids light up when one of their presents really struck a chord. My folks were very thoughtful. They sacrificed their own wants to save enough money to get us kids things that really meant something to us. And they weren't always expensive, material things. My very first dog, who came to live with me when I was eight years old, was a present from Santa.

So was a trip to the 1995 Rose Bowl which is an experience I'll never forget. While my dad would certainly have loved to go watch the Rose Bowl game in person, he got more joy out of sending my brother and me to Pasadena to watch it together. Hearing our stories and seeing our reactions meant more to him than anything else.

Fast forward many years, when something that happened helped me understand why giving more than receiving meant so much to my parents. I was at a conference in Palm Springs and happened to have the same server at the hotel bar and restaurant the entire week I was there. As a former bartender/bouncer/server myself, I tend to be quite friendly with wait staff, and he and I shared many good conversations. As it turned out, the man I'll call Marcos was originally from Mexico City. He and his wife were separated and shared custody of their eight-year-old daughter who was, in his words, "the light of my life."

At this conference there was a trade show with many booths and displays that had giveaways as a way to get your business card from you. The idea, of course, is if you drop your card in this box you're entered to win this iPad, and now I (the guy manning the booth) have a bunch of potential clients' business cards to show my boss when I get back to my office so he knows I wasn't goofing off the entire time.

I was excited to learn that I'd won a portable DVD player in one of the trade show drawings. It was delivered to me while I was enjoying a drink at the hotel bar that evening. Marcos noticed it and asked me about it. As I explained how I acquired that DVD player, I could tell he was jealous of my prize. In our conversations, we never got into personal financial details, but my guess is that if he was a full-time server at a hotel bar and a single parent, he certainly didn't have a whole lot of cash lying around for extras. Even for his daughter.

"Marcos," I eventually said, "what would your daughter think about having something like this just for herself?"

"Josh, my friend, if she was lucky enough to have something like this, it would mean the world to her. It would be like Christmas."

I handed him the DVD player. "Well, Marcos, Merry Christmas. You take this home to your daughter. Don't tell her how you got it, but make sure she knows you got it for her because you care that much for her. And thanks for being such a great server this week."

The gesture almost made him cry. He even refused to accept it until I told him I was going to leave it on the table. If he didn't take it, I added, someone else would.

How thankful he was, and it was such a small and easy gesture on my part for such a huge payoff. That DVD player that I'd won meant way more to that little girl than it ever would have to me.

As I think about it now, my giving the DVD player to Marcos for his daughter was like my parents being able to watch my excitement when I went to the Rose Bowl. It meant the world to them. And to me.

So I guess what they say is true: *"'Tis better to give than to receive."*

Which is also true in running.

I thought running the Boston marathon would never be bettered by any other race I would ever run from that point forward. "No way it could get better than this," I told myself.

I was wrong.

Several family members and friends had come to Boston to cheer me on. One was my sister Laurie, a marathoner herself. Laurie had come close to qualifying previously, but she'd never really made a conscious effort in her training to actually qualify. Now she was so captivated by the entire experience (as was everyone in my group, the non-runners included) that after the race she looked me square in the eye and told me she was going to qualify and come back and run the race next year.

"I'm going to do it," she told me. "But I'll need your help."

Laurie is ten years older than I am, so I was pretty young during her high school years and when she left home for college. But the age gap never fazed her. She used to take me into the student seating section for the Friday-night football games. (How many high schoolers do you know would take their seven-year-old brother with them to hang out with their friends?) I remember one day when I being was bullied so badly by a much bigger kid in the neighborhood I stormed back into the house bawling my eyes out. When she found out what happened she was so furious she marched right down to the kid's house, knocked on the door, and tore that kid a new backside until he promised he would never mess with me again. I'm pretty sure I saw him pee a little bit standing there on his own front porch. And you know what? He never messed with me again. Never.

When I first decided to try to run a half marathon, my first call was to Laurie to ask for her advice. I also asked her to be my first running coach and mentor. Boy, was she flattered at the opportunity to mentor her little brother.

So when she asked for *my* help? I was so honored. There wasn't a chance I'd refuse. Not a question.

Laurie named the coming October's race in Columbus, Ohio as her target for qualifying for Boston. She and I had run that race together a few years earlier (it was my first Boston qualifier) and considering how flat the course is and the fact that it's the town she was living in, we agreed that it was a solid choice.

Next, she introduced track work and hills into her training and diversified her cross training to the extent that she completed her first half Ironman that June. (For non-runners reading this, an Ironman consists of a 2.4 mile swim, a 112 mile bike ride, and a 26.2 mile run. A half ironman is half the distances of all three, consecutively and in that order.) Her theory was that diversifying her exercise would increase her overall fitness and ultimately make her a faster runner, allowing her to shave enough off of her personal best marathon time in order to notch her first Boston qualifier. She was committed to making her qualifying time, but was still convinced that without my help, she had no shot at success.

I agreed to run part of the Columbus race with her, but because of several factors, my legs just weren't ready to run a full 26.2 miles at any pace. I was stuck finding a balance between minimizing my own mileage covered while at the same time maximizing the support I gave my sister. To complicate matters, I had coached another runner through her first half marathon in June and we had her ready to run in Columbus. Now she, too, was requesting my support for as much of the race as possible.

This was going to be tricky.

We found a spot on the course around Mile 15 ½ where I could meet up with my sister to run the final 10+ miles alongside her. To clarify, because simply jumping in for the last ten miles of a race is usually against the rules, to be fair to the race, its organizers, and the other runners, I registered and paid for the full marathon registration. That made me a full, legal participant. By rule, since I didn't run the entire race and cross the checkpoints (each runner will have a chip somewhere on their person and will cross certain checkpoints along most organized races), then I would be disqualified and receive a "Did Not Finish" from the race officials. Which was fine. I didn't care about that. I was there to help my sister, and as long as I was a fully-paid participant, I wasn't breaking any rules by jumping in part-way along the course.

Her qualifying time was 3:45, and I knew her training times put her right on the bubble for that, so when I got to the sidewalk to wait for her, I was surprised to see her turn the corner on the heels of the 3:40 pace group. She was ahead of schedule. I jumped right in to run with her.

"How are you feeling, dude?" I asked her.

"Dude, you have a big job ahead of you."

We call each other dude, by the way. Always have.

She then explained to me that she'd come out a bit too quick, so although she was in good shape as far as time, she was figuring on struggling and slowing down for the home stretch.

I did some math in my head. If she kept up a nine-minute per mile pace for the final 10 ½ miles, we would be celebrating a Boston qualifier. At first, that pace seemed reasonable, as we were trucking along at a sub 8:30 pace. I monitored closely on my GPS watch. (Laurie didn't have a GPS watch of her own. She still doesn't. Which reinforces my claims that you don't need fancy gear to succeed in running.) As she suspected she would, she slowed down. The 8:30 overall pace she'd kept up for our first three or four miles started slipping. Each time I looked at my watch, I grew more and more nervous. 8:30 turned into 8:35. Then it slipped to 8:40. Soon it was 8:45. When I saw that we were now at an 8:50 overall pace at about Mile 20, I knew she needed a bit of a kick in the ass.

"All right, dude," I told her, "here's the situation. Your pace has been slipping, and we're now up over 8:50 per mile. You're still ahead of pace, but you can't afford to keep slowing like this. We need to pick up this pace if you want to have a shot at this thing."

"I'm doing the best I can," she muttered.

Not in a mean way. More of a "I can barely see straight I'm so tired and now you want me to run *faster*?"

Which she didn't actually need to tell me. I knew she was struggling. Her sudden halt to our conversations, her cursing out loud at even the slightest bit of incline, and the changes in her breathing and running posture had already shown me she was fading. But she was six miles away from punching her ticket to Boston. She'd kick herself if she slacked now.

So I came up with a game plan consisting of an old trick I'd taught myself. "All right, dude," I said, "here's what we're gonna do. Quit doing math in your head. Because right now you have six total miles left, and that seems at this point to be an impossible task to complete at this pace. So we're not going to run six miles. Or even two miles. We're just going to run *one mile*. Get to Mile 21 keeping up a solid 8:50 pace, and then we'll take it from there and see how you're feeling. But right now, that's all I want you to focus on. *Run one more mile*."

"Okay, I'll try." That was all she could muster.

Holding a steady pace, we got to Mile 21. I congratulated her and instructed her to do the same thing again: just one more mile. Just run one more mile at this pace. That's all I wanted her to focus on. Once we got that second mile taken care of, we'd figure out the rest.

Despite her struggles, she seemed to be able to keep her focus on running a mile at a time. By Mile 25, her overall pace since I'd joined her had steadied at 8:50/mile. I kept turning around and running backwards to make sure the 3:45 pace group wasn't on our heels. Every time I looked, they were nowhere in sight.

(Another point of clarity for non runners and less experienced runners. Many races will have pace leaders for both the half marathon and full marathon distances. These leaders will typically hold signs or carry balloons that indicate a certain time they plan to finish the race in. Those pace leaders are very seasoned, well-trained runners who can help pace you to exactly the time listed on their sign or balloon. Laurie and other runners that day who were trying to finish the marathon in a time of 3:45 could follow the designated and marked 3:45 pace leader. A side note to this clarification: I accomplished one of my Boston qualifying times at the Virginia Beach Marathon. It was a very windy day, so our two pace leaders had recruited two of their running buddies to come and help them pace. They huddled all of us runners together before the race began and coached us to have everyone tuck in behind the four of them, single file, any time there was a head wind. They were thus essentially blocking the wind for us and letting us draft and save precious energy along the course. Which was *crucial*, as that happened to be an overly windy day that presented us with several nasty headwinds later in the race. It's a very generous, giving gesture which falls right in line with the life lesson highlighted in this chapter.)

About half a mile from the finish line, I began celebrating under the assumption that I needed to celebrate for her since she had no energy left to do much of anything.

"Unless you get struck by lightning or hit by a car," I told her, "this is happening. You're about to qualify for Boston."

When we got to the home stretch, the crowd at the finish line was going crazy. I give credit to the citizens of Columbus for providing great fan support during that race.

Before the race I'd had a shirt made which said something like, *"Helping pace my sister to run her very first Boston qualifier"* with an arrow pointing right at her. (I had to ask her beforehand on which side of her she would prefer me to run so I could have the arrow pointed in her direction.) You can imagine how crazy the crowd and fellow runners went when they read my shirt.

We crossed the finish line with about a minute to spare. My sister had just qualified for the Boston Marathon. Very big deal. I gave her a giant hug. We still have a picture of her crossing the finish line with her arms raised in celebration and me by her side in my custom made shirt throwing a huge fist pump through the air.

I could tell she was exhausted. I wanted to hang out with her to celebrate, but my other runner was still out on the course and probably still needed a bit of a pick-me-up. The only way I was going to be able to get to her was to run back up the course, essentially double backing and running the course backwards, until I met up with her.

So I congratulated Laurie one more time, grabbed a bottle of water, and started hoofing it back up the course. I spotted the other runner I was coaching around Mile 23. I turned around and started running alongside her. Because she was a first-timer, I worked with her the same way I had with Laurie. Everyone could see my fist-pumping and my clapping and cheering as she and I ran along the home stretch toward the finish line. We crossed the line and I gave my second giant hug of the day. What an awesome experience that race was.

Then I looked at my watch and chuckled. I had run a total of 17.44 miles. So much for keeping my mileage low that day. But that didn't really matter. Both of my runners had met their goals.

Qualify for Boston: check.

Finish the race without vomiting or dying: check.

Although Laurie continues to insist to this day that she couldn't have done it without me, they certainly both could have done it without my help. But what an amazing experience it was to be a part of accomplishing their major life goal. Getting to cross that finish line with both of them that day tops any other experience I've ever had in running.

It was better than the first time I crossed the finish line.

It was better than the first time I qualified for Boston.

It was better than when I ran Boston.

Helping, coaching, and mentoring other runners is amazingly gratifying. It is, I have found, more satisfying than anything you can do in your own running. And most coaches and teachers will say the same thing. Watching one of their players or students learn and grow and accomplish something due to your help gives them more of a sense of accomplishment than anything they have ever done as an individual.

Being a mentor or a good boss is the same thing. Helping people is in our nature. And it feels great when we're able to do it. A friend of mine has a sister-in-law who spends most of her running time helping others. While she has qualified for Boston multiple times, she prefers to spend her racing time helping others finish. She also runs alongside many first-timers, whatever their pace may be, so she can support them throughout the race. She would rather lend a helping hand to support others than worry about her own times and pace.

What an outstanding attitude and approach that is. The world of running needs more folks like that. As does the world in general.

An old friend recently told me a story about a 5k she ran near the town she lives in. Typically, she tends to rush to the race, run it, then immediately head back home, but for some reason on this particular day she was inspired to hang around the finish line and cheer the other runners on. She watched two middle-school boys toward the back of the pack cross the finish line together. One of them had his hands on the shoulders of his running mate and friend. After looking closely, she saw that the second boy was blind. His friend had run the entire way to guide him along the course, allowing him to participate. Seeing such generosity is inspiring to both runners and non-runners alike.

Life lesson learned: *Pay it forward by helping others.* You'll be amazed at what you get in return.

9

Be a Better Person

> Oh, horseshit, Dottie. Of course it's hard. It's supposed to be hard. If it were easy, everyone would do it. The hard…is what makes it great.
> —Jimmy Dugan, played by Tom Hanks
> in *A League of Their Own*

Perfection is something that most of us strive for but nobody, ever, in the history of the world, has achieved. To err is human, as Alexander Pope wrote two hundred years ago, and life has always seemed to be one long saga of making mistakes, hopefully learning from those mistakes, and making fewer, less drastic mistakes as we grow and mature.

Running is not an exception to that reality. Our running lives are littered with mistakes that range from being arrogant and bragging about our running to overtraining and ultimately injuring ourselves. Just like other people, we runners try to learn from our mistakes (and the mistakes of others) to minimize our own, but no matter how hard we try, we still make running mistakes. We have to recognize what those mistakes are and try to be just a bit better at not repeating them the next time.

Runners have different motivations for why we run. People exercise for various reasons. Typically our motivations for exercising in general to running in particular tend to change as the other parts of our lives change.

When I first started running, my motivation was to simply prove that I could do it. I felt like I had to prove to myself and others that Josh Wackler could run 13.1, and eventually 26.2 miles. But now my motivation has shifted. Now I run for a different reason.

Readers, just like all of you, I am not perfect. While my parents instilled a strong sense of morals and ethics in me, I still fail every day. I fall short every day of the man I could and should be. In fact, when I started making a list of ways in which I fail and areas in which

I am not perfect to include in this chapter, I quickly realized that the list was too long to try to fit into a book.

I'm not trying to point out that I'm a bad guy. Hopefully that's not the case. But I can tell you beyond a shadow of a doubt that every night when my head hits the pillow, I think of a significant list of things I could have done different that day. I could have called my mother. I could have smiled more. Yes, plenty of improvements to make. You get the picture.

And while running is certainly not the silver bullet cure-all, I feel like my running has helped me significantly reduce the length and severity of my list of imperfections. There is a history of addiction, overweight issues, high blood pressure, high cholesterol and diabetes in my family. Running has, so far, helped me steer clear of all of these maladies. It gives me a healthy outlet to deal with stress and fatigue. And yes, while you may think I'm crazy, physical exercise does actually increase your energy level in the long term.

I don't need running just because it makes me physically feel better and more energized throughout the day. I don't need running just because it gives me an outlet for daily stresses and relief from them. I don't need running just because it allows me to get away from the rest of the world and be with my own thoughts for an hour every day. I don't need running just because it teaches me about focus, discipline, hard work, commitment. and dealing with adversity.

I don't need running just because of the sense of accomplishment it gives me, like having learned a great deal from my mistakes.

And I don't need running just because it gives me an opportunity to help others.

I don't need running just because of any of the reasons I just gave.

I need running because of all of them.

Training for and running marathons is physically difficult. It's really hard. But it's supposed to be hard. The hard is what makes it great. Most people probably can run a marathon, but few people ever will run a marathon. That's because it's just too hard. But the challenge is what some of us crave.

The challenge of seeking perfection is a losing battle, but we will continue to fight that battle because we constantly want to improve ourselves. As runners, we also constantly want to improve our running.

Coming back full circle to the connection between why I run and all of my imperfections, figuring out why I run becomes pretty simple.

I run to be a better person.

10

Destination vs. Journey

My fifth and final year of college (yes, I was a "victory lap" student) was probably my favorite year. My fondest memory of that year was the Insight Bowl in Phoenix, Arizona, when my beloved Oregon State Beavers beat the Notre Dame Fighting Irish in a bowl game for the second time in five years. I attended the game with four buddies, all of whom were fellow bouncers/bartenders at the most popular pub in the Corvallis, Oregon, area. We bought our tickets together and made the long drive from sleepy Corvallis to Phoenix. The game was amazing. Watching your college team beat Notre Dame is a great experience.

But the game wasn't the highlight.

The road trip was.

Although now, years later, I can describe it as a fond, funny memory, at the time it was the worst road trip of our lives. The following is a list of situations we encountered on the round trip. I'm not exaggerating.

1) A blizzard in Northern California and a road closure there resulting in our being delayed and sleeping in the car in a snow-filled parking lot.
2) A windstorm that led to a dust storm in Southern California resulting in our being delayed.
3) Flash flooding in Phoenix resulted in our being delayed.
4) Flooding in the Bay Area on our way back home made us divert to Highway 101 rather than staying on I-5, which led to another delay.
5) A rockslide we encountered in Northern California on the way home resulted in two blown tires and two shattered rims. And another delay.

A road trip that is supposed to take eighteen hours took us twenty-four hours on the way down to Phoenix and over thirty hours on the way back home. None of us could believe how awful our luck was, We couldn't wait until that road trip ended.

But as I look back on it today, all those delays are what made the trip more memorable. In other words, the trip was memorable because of the journey itself. Not the destination.

That's because all those difficulties we ran into make for a great story now. A story that years later I'm still telling people. And the five of us still reminisce about it whenever we see each other.

But running isn't focused on a destination. Sometimes people get so focused on one particular day and one particular race that they see it as one single goal and one single destination. Running is so much more than that.

Reaching your destination can do more for you than I realized when I decided to run my first race. Running will teach you discipline and focus. How to be committed to something. How to overcome obstacles and move forward despite adversity.

Running has taught me so much more about life than I ever realized it could. Most of our life lessons happen during the journey. Not just at the destination.

Before I ran the Boston Marathon for the first time, I posted on my blog and wrote about my fear of feeling empty after I'd run the Big Kahuna. I was projecting a sort of "all right, now what?" attitude. Once you've run Boston, I thought, there isn't really anything left to do, and I was worried about an apparent struggle with where to run after the marathon. Where could I go next?

Like so many things in my life…I was wrong.

After that first Boston race, I was more energized than ever to keep running. Even after experiencing what is probably the most amazing course and crowd that exists in the entire world, I was then—and still am—more excited than ever. More enamored with the sport. I have developed an obsession with running.

I tell people all the time that the hard part about running a marathon isn't running a marathon per se. It's the 180 days leading up to running the marathon. It's like the hardest part about being a major league starting pitcher. It's not the thirty days a year when you're pitching. It's the other 335 days of the year when you are recovering, training, working out, and studying your opponents and their weaknesses.

Was running the Boston Marathon one of the most striking and amazing experiences of my life? You bet it was. Is Boston a destination? Sure it is. A magnificent one. Both the race and the city itself. Was my qualifying for and running a destination? Not even close. It was a long, difficult, sometimes heart-breaking journey. And that journey is ongoing.

It's ongoing because there are so many other things to accomplish on this life journey called running. There are other races to run. Other runners to cheer on. Other beginners to help get started.

The reason Boston is so prestigious to us runners is because of how difficult it is to get there. (In order to qualify to run the Boston Marathon, you first must find and register to run a full marathon, which is a Boston Qualifier certified race. Most races these days are certified, but I suggest you thoroughly read the website to make sure. Once you have registered, you must finish the 26.2 distance in under a time designated by the Boston Athletic Association, which varies depending on your gender and age. Women's times in each age group are thirty more minutes than men's, and as you move up in age groups, you will be allowed anywhere between five and fifteen additional minutes with that next age group. The Association has had to lower the times several times recently because average running times are becoming faster, so this could change again. As an example, at the time I'm typing this, a twenty-six-year-old male would have to run a BQ certified race in under three hours in order to qualify. Which is roughly 6:50 minutes per mile. Yowza...) There is no denying that running the course itself is difficult. While it is a net downhill course, the hills between miles 16 and 21 make it one of the more grueling courses.

It's put up on a sort of pedestal, though, because it's the most prestigious race in the U.S. I live in Nashville, and many musical acts will say that they put the Ryman concert venue (the original Grand Ole Opry) on a pedestal because it's such an iconic and historic venue. Similar concepts. What is significant about the Boston Marathon is the journey it takes to get to Boston and to the race. Once you're there, you're there. You can run it as fast or as slow as you want to. But getting there is like that long road trip to Phoenix my buddies and I took during which nothing seemed to go right.

In running, as in nearly everything else, there will be times of triumph and happiness. Also times of heartbreak. You might decide all the trouble it takes to get there just isn't worth it. Or you decide you'd rather give up than continue to try and fail again. There are days when you think there's no way in hell you'll ever meet your goal. Your emotions will bounce up and down. Doubt. Remorse. Exhaustion. Helplessness. Regret. Satisfaction. Happiness. Pride. Excitement.

All of these are emotions that are almost sure to flood you while you're training to run a race. Good or bad, all these feelings will eventually turn you into a better person. A better sibling. A better parent. A better coworker.

While the race itself will teach us a lot about life, what really has taught me these lessons and made me a better person are the days leading up to the race.

The training.

The journey.

I have heard a lot of runners, even so-called experts, talk about race day being a huge physical struggle. They tell us that the 26.2 miles is eighty percent physical and twenty percent mental. Or they give some other arbitrary set of percentages. I disagree with the conventional wisdom. In fact, I look at it the opposite way: race day is eighty percent mental and only twenty percent physical.

Race day to me is a *mental battle*. Not a physical one.

When people hear me say that, they're usually ready to have me committed. That's because one thing for certain is that during a long race, at some point you are going to hurt. And when I say hurt, I mean HURT. You may ask yourself what in the hell ever made you think that this race was a good idea. Your legs are feeling like hot pokers being beaten by a huge ball peen hammer. Physically, you'll be totally worn down and more exhausted than maybe you've ever been.

And that's not the really hard part.

If you have ever stood at the finish line of a marathon and watched while people crossed, you'll know that it's fairly common to see someone who just physically shuts down and can't even reach the finish line. It happens at every race. But those folks are the exception, not the rule. And that shutdown is usually a result of either hot weather or insufficient training.

If you have trained properly and stuck to your training plan, your body will hold up. You may not finish in your desired time, but you'll get there before your body shuts itself down. It will keep going and keep running.

But only if your grit makes it.

While your legs will keep moving and your arms will keep pumping, the trick is to be mentally tough enough to make sure your brain keeps telling your legs and arms to keep going. That's why the truly difficult part of the race becomes what I call a lack of accountability.

You ask yourself, "If I don't finish this race, am I going to lose my job? Is my family going to disown me? Other than anguish, are there truly any consequences to my just giving up? What if I just don't finish? Am I accountable to anyone besides myself?"

What's stopping you from slacking off or giving up? There isn't any accountability other than to yourself. So the race actually becomes a mental struggle.

It's your brain. And how tough your brain is makes all the difference in the world.

And when your mental toughness keeps making you put one foot in front of the other and you cross that finish line, your sense of satisfaction at finishing that damn race will be thanks to all that you have invested in preparing for that race and everything you went through during that journey.

Had I just flown to Phoenix, gone to the bowl game, and flown home, the days wouldn't have been nearly as memorable as they were. It's because of all the trying situations we were put in that I'll remember it forever. Whenever I think about that trip up and down the West Coast and into Arizona, I can't help but smile. The memories of that journey will always make me smile.

The journey to get there is what made it so special.

The journey to achieve 26.2 miles what makes the marathon special.

As in life.

Life lesson learned: *Life is a journey. Not a destination.*

11

Slow Down to Go Faster

Whenever a person sets a goal to run a race of any distance, the most obvious thing they need to plan for is the running itself. To get your body in shape to run considerably further than you are physically able to run today, it should be obvious that a slow increase in both distance and frequency is going to be required if you want to reach your goal.

But there is a second key factor that, if neglected, can spell disaster to your training. We all have friends and/or family members who fail to exercise for one reason or another. For example, let's say that one of those folks who neglects his exercise and hasn't run or done any kind of physical activity for over a year decides to go out in his neighborhood tonight and run a mile just as fast as he can. He will finish that mile in whatever time is appropriate to him. Tomorrow night he decides to go out and do the same thing, running a mile as fast as he can. Chances are, the guy's body and muscles are already pretty stiff and sore from that first night's fast mile. So on the second night, while he might complete the mile again, it would take longer. Let's say he goes out for a run on the third night. He's aiming for a hard, fast run. But the truth is, he will probably hobble and limp and struggle through most of the mile. He might not even be able to finish.

If stupidity prevails and the guy tries a fourth night in a row, my guess is that he won't even be able to make it as far as the starting line because his body would feel so beat up that the chances of his completing that fourth mile are minimal.

Sometimes people get one sided with exercise. We get it stuck in our head that if X amount of exercise is good, then exercising five times that amount is five times as good. The more we exercise, that is, the better shape we'll be in, so we say to ourselves, "I'm going to come out of the gate with my hair on fire." But what people usually forget is that second key factor: runners need to rest. Resting is just as important as running.

A comprehensive examination of the anatomy and physiology of the human body and how running and resting work on the body would requires more space than this book permits. The best way I can describe how your body becomes more fit is that you have to hurt it.

Essentially, when you tear your muscles and injure your insides ever so slightly, your ever-efficient body repairs itself. When it repairs itself and comes back, it comes back a bit stronger and more efficient than it was before. Then the cycle repeats.

But if you don't ever allow your body to take time to rest and heal itself, that vitally important aspect of rest and repair is neglected, and you'll never reach your fitness goals. In fact, you're likely to remain injured.

Which is why we runners need to find that delicate balance between not running enough and running too much. While all of our bodies are different, I have found that my large frame starts seeing diminishing returns once I eclipse forty-five to fifty miles in a given week. While some elite athletes and Olympic hopefuls can train twice a day and run eighty to 130 miles per week, that kind of pounding on my legs with my frame will break me down. My point is that all of us need to find that delicate balance and that whatever that balance ends up being is different for everyone. That's going to take some trial and error on your part. But always err on the side of being conservative when you're first starting out. When in doubt, less is more.

But even Olympic runners understand that rest is necessary. Some of them take one day a week to rest, and they certainly don't run eighty to 130 miles per week all year long. They get to their peak mileage while preparing for a specific event, then cut back for a time to let their body recuperate. This is what is referred to as "tapering."

I once read a comment by a very famous American marathoner that he stays completely away from any exercise at all for two weeks after a marathon in which he went full out. He knows his body needs rest after he's put it through the grueling punishment of a full marathon.

It's a policy that I have decided to adopt. Sometimes, of course, it's difficult to convince ourselves that we need the rest and that more miles aren't always better. We have to make a strategic decision to occasionally step away from running so we can come back to the next race refreshed, both mentally and physically.

People need this same lesson with their profession, career, or day job. Too often, we let our job define who we are as a person. We also let our job get in the way of things like family and recreation which should have a higher priority. Like our four-day runner above, we fail to schedule time to step away and rest so we can come back refreshed.

"But," I hear you saying, "going on vacation just isn't worth it to me because I'm just way too busy and when I come back, I'm backed up with work. So I would just rather not take a vacation."

We've all heard people say this, and some of us have probably even said it ourselves. In my opinion, that is the exact opposite of what we should do. We should take our vacations. We need to rest, physically, mentally, emotionally.

I sometimes say to the folks I have supervised, "I don't want to get any work-related calls while you're out of the office. I don't want to see you respond to any work-related emails over the weekend or while you're on vacation. The work," I add, "will still be here when you get back. Right now, you need to take care of yourself and stay away from work." Sometimes they listen. But oftentimes they don't.

And me? I always make it a point to go on several vacations, just to get away. Some of them are ten-day trips across the pond, and some are three-day weekends just down the road. Even if things seem hectic and backed-up at work, I don't let anything get in the way of my vacations because I know how much more efficient I'll be once I come back.

Just as I believe I don't have enough time *not* to work out because of how much more efficient I am during the rest of the day when I consistently exercise, I can't afford *not* to go on vacation because of how much more efficient I am during the other fifty weeks of the year. Sometimes my life needs to slow down. That's when I go to the gym or out on the roads so that the rest of my life can speed up. Sometimes the slowing down means taking a vacation away from everything and has the same healing effect. And is the week when I come back to my job unusually hectic while I'm trying to catch up? Sure it is. But it's certainly not the end of the world. I always get caught up.

I have learned that when you take care of yourself first and make sure you're healthy and stress-free by giving those things which are important to you a higher priority, you eventually become more efficient at your job. You're also better to be around and work with.

Sometimes my running needs to slow down. I need to rest so that my running can eventually go faster. Of course running requires working your ass off and then resting until you can go back to working your ass off. So does life.

Life lesson learned: *Sometimes you need to slow down to go faster.*

12

Motivation

Citius, Altius, Fortius. It means faster, higher, stronger. It's been the motto for the Olympics for the last 2500 years. But it doesn't mean faster, higher and stronger than who you are competing against. Just faster, higher, stronger.
—Bill Bowerman, played by Donald Sutherland,
in *Without Limits*,
a movie about runner Steve Prefontaine

Runners can be labeled a strange bunch. Not entirely, but mostly, because if you run for long enough, you develop a capacity to have no shame whatsoever. We do strange things like carry water bottles everywhere we go, we dress in clothes that make us look like a human-sized walking highlighter, we relieve ourselves anywhere we can during races, and we order and consume two entrees to ourselves during any given business lunch.

Sometimes I wonder what goes through the heads of non-runners when they observe runners as we do such things. Or even what goes through their heads when they're just watching me running down the road. Do they ask themselves what would motivate a person to just take off running down the sidewalk for fun?

I suppose, comparatively speaking, watching a runner run is like watching a high energy dog when he's turned loose in a big field or yard. I get a high level of amusement watching dogs because they run around like maniacs. There's no pattern in their running, and to say those dogs run circular "laps" would be an unfair blow to geometry. Sometimes they run in a figure 8, while other times they run in a zig-zag pattern. And other times they run in no discernible pattern at all. But whatever pattern they happen to prefer at any given moment, they just run. And run. And run some more.

But not without breaks. They'll be running like maniacs, and suddenly, without warning, they'll stop dead in their tracks to stare at you with a tongue hanging out of one side or the other of their mouth, staring you down. It's as if the dog is saying, "Um, hello? Why aren't you running, too?" After a few seconds of said intense stare, the dog's limited attention span has been more than maxed out. So then the dog barks as if to say, "Okay, fine, be that way. But you have no idea what you're missing!" Then he takes off again in the same charming form, tongue waving in the wind, drool flying every which way.

I love dogs and I love watching dogs do this. It gives me a lot of amusement for several reasons. Like people during the running parts of their lives, dogs seem to lack any kind of concern for the judgment of other dogs (or people). Dogs want you to love them, and runners want to finish their run. That's all. Outside of that, we really couldn't care less about your judging eyes making fun of my sunglasses, which don't happen to match my shorts that day.

I watch my own dog, Clodfelter the Boxer, run like this nearly every day and say to myself, "Look at that crazy dog! He's running around the yard in figure eights with drool all over his body and grass stained feet. What a silly dog!" But does he care? Fat chance.

They say that dogs often resemble their owners. I suppose this could be true with Clodfelter and me with the indifference to human judgment. My guess is that it's not rare for non-runners to see me running down the street and wonder what that big idiot is doing dressed like that, sweating all over himself, and speeding around on these busy streets. I just don't care. Judge me all you want, but I'll stay over here out of earshot. Running.

People could benefit greatly in many situations from letting go of their worry about what other people think of them, at least to a certain extent. If you don't care whether people judged you or not when you robbed that bank, that's your prerogative, but the courts are probably going to frown at bank-robbing.

Lesson from a dog and a runner: *just let go*. So what if someone thinks you look silly? Who cares? Do you remember when you were a kid and ran around the yard for no particular reason at all? I can't say for sure why you did that, but my guess is you did it (a) because it was fun and (b) that you had no concern whatsoever with what people thought about you while you were running. Just like our dogs, kids really don't care if people think we look silly. We ran when we were kids because it felt good and we had fun doing it.

People tend to over-analyze everything. We tend to look for a complicated answer or explanation to even simple questions, usually when a simple answer will do just fine. We can try to get deep and psychoanalyze why dogs run around the yard. Or why all kids and adult runners run. I'm sure someone could even come up with a lengthy thesis for their master's or doctoral program on human brain function and how it impacts why we run.

In my humble opinion, answering the question about why my dog and why most kids run around that yard is the same answer to many other questions. The answer is that there is no answer.

Why do you prefer redheads over blondes? Why do I love eating yogurt but refuse to eat cottage cheese? Why can a person stare at a campfire for hours at a time without getting bored? Why does Clodfelter love playing with and eating grapefruits but is terrified of my broom, which sends him cowering and shaking into the basement every time I sweep?

We just do. That's simply the way it is.

Yes, we have a difficult time coming up with a more in-depth, complex explanation to questions like these.

But do we really need one?

As I get more years under my running belt, I struggle to answer the motivation question because the premise behind the question still confuses me. Clodfelter the Boxer and the younger you didn't need to find motivation. You just ran around whenever you had the chance because you enjoyed it. But later in life, people need a more logical answer. This confuses me because a simple answer is more than enough.

Does it bother you when you climb a single flight of stairs and you find yourself noticeably winded? Do you enjoy hearing compliments from people who ask you if you've lost weight or tell you how great you look in those pants? Do you actually prefer staying at home and watching that reality show on TV instead of working a sweat up during a good, hard run around your neighborhood? Or getting some laps in the pool, or whatever else your preferred form of exercise is?

It's no secret that different people have different motivations for exercising. Maybe it's a simple fitness thing. Maybe it's a stress reliever. Maybe it's a way to escape from your job, your screaming kids, the bills, and whatever other stresses in your life. Maybe it's a way to help keep yourself focused on things you do when you're not running. Maybe your doctor—or that heart attack—scared the hell out of you and you decided to take up running. Maybe you run to get yourself through a tough time.

Or maybe you run to remember a fallen loved one. I'll never forget my experience running the Oklahoma City Memorial Marathon, which was named as a way to remember those who died in the Oklahoma City terrorist bombings in 1995. Part of the marathon course overlaps the 5k course, and every 5k runner when I was there was wearing a race shirt with this on the back: *Running to remember* _____. In the blank, of course, was the hand-written name of an individual unexpectedly lost in that American tragedy.

What struck me even more than the names was that every runner I saw was struggling through the 5k, walking or running at a snail's pace and wincing with every step. Yet even through their difficulties, each runner I passed managed to thank me for running to remember their fallen loved one. I wanted to stop and hug each one of them and say that it was I who should be thanking them. If that doesn't get you choked up, nothing will.

I was also once schooled by a young college student on his own ways of motivating himself. As he spoke, my smile kept growing. He was telling me that no matter what happened in his life with homework, tests, family, other people doing stupid things, or whatever else was going on, he could always run. Because, he said, "Out here, it's just me and God. And I don't have to answer to anyone but him and myself." I sure wish I'd had that level of insight at age nineteen.

It seems like there's a constant battle of wits between those of us who run and those of us who don't run. We ask each other the same questions:

Why do you run?

Why don't you run?

The best answer I can give, and I admittedly have struggled to find, boils down to one simple concept. My sense of accomplishment and pride when I cross the finish line of a long race rivals anything else I have ever done in my entire existence.

When you're running, you're thinking about everything you have invested in that race. You think about the blisters. The ice baths. The 4 a.m. and midnight runs. The heartbreak of an injury and the satisfaction of a great run. Getting your training in despite rain, sleet, cold, hot, humid, or any other non-ideal conditions. There's a pretty good chance that you've shed blood, sweat, and tears while you were training. Sometimes all three simultaneously. You ran through a flu or a head cold. Maybe an excruciatingly sore back.

And then you come to one simple fact: *I did it.* I stared all that adversity right in the face and I succeeded despite it all. And if I set out to run this race and was successful, I can set out to do anything and be successful.

Crossing the finish line is an amazing feeling. It's better than that slice of homemade cheesecake after a great meal. Better than your favorite ice cold beer on a hot day. It's better than that feeling that went all the way down to the pit in your stomach when you had your first crush on the third-grade playground.

It makes you realize that all of those sacrifices were worth it. Sometimes you may have doubted they were worth it. You also doubted your training plan. Doubted that your peers were really encouraging you. Doubted yourself.

But cross that finish line and all doubt disappears.

Completing a 26.2 mile race is one of the most difficult things a person will do in their entire life. It's also one of the most rewarding things they'll do in their entire life.

What I'm trying to get to here is an apology to those folks who asked for guidance in running and asked me the motivation question and got a sub-par answer. Why do I run is a difficult question for me to wrap my head around because I don't really have to answer it for myself. The best way I can tackle a good answer is to remember that never once, under any conditions other than having injured myself, have I gone out for a run and after completion had the thought, "Boy—I sure wish I hadn't done that."

Life lesson learned: *Those things in life which give you the most reward are typically the most difficult to accomplish.*

Isn't that motivation enough?

13

Dream Big

As young kids, we are dreamers by human nature. We imagine we're astronauts, that we have wings and can fly, that we're as strong as He-Man and as fast as Wile E. Coyote.

I was no different. I can still remember watching the Atlanta Braves on TV almost every day they played. They were always televised on TBS, so it was either watch the Braves or don't watch baseball at all. I would stand in front of the TV, bat in hand, get into a batting stance, and try to mimic Chipper Jones, Andruw Jones, and David Justice, to name just three players. I also imitated them with a glove while they were out in the field. And I replayed every move of what was probably the greatest pitching staff I have ever seen: Tom Glavine, John Smoltz, Greg Maddux, and Steve Avery.

I believed, I *knew*, that I would be out there one day as a big leaguer and that I would be thanking those same players for their help and inspiration. And my dreams didn't stop there. I was convinced that I was going to be the first person in the history of professional sports to be a professional athlete in the three primary American sports: baseball, basketball, and football. I wrote about it in a fifth grade assignment, which was to write my own future autobiography, telling the story of my yet-to-be-lived life.

Being the youngest of four, I was no stranger to being teased and picked on. My three older siblings frequently disagreed with my professional aspirations in three sports. Whenever she heard them, our mom, being the amazing mother she still is, always got very angry with them when she heard their comments about how unrealistic my aspirations were and what a stupid dream it was.

"All three of you need to cut that crap out right now," she always told them. "If he wants to do it, you let him believe he can do it. And I don't want to hear any different from any of you."

Life itself, along with growing up in the real world, tends to squash our dreams and grind down our belief in ourselves and our capability to dream big. Obviously, many of the dreams we had as kids are biologically and physically impossible. Humans do not evolve into creatures of flight and spider webs will not mysteriously start shooting out of our wrists. But other, more realistic, dreams and goals also fall out of our grasp because we fail too many times and are told often enough by others that something just isn't going to happen. We hear the nay-sayers so often that we eventually start to believe them and accept what they say as fact and reality. Like, I didn't get accepted into medical school, so I guess I wasn't destined to be a doctor. Yale turned me down, so I guess my dream to go to school there was shot. Mr. Jones gave me a C in calculus, so I suppose he was right—I'm just not cut out to be an engineer.

I can't even run a half mile, so there is no way in the world I can run 26.2 miles.

I am forever grateful to my mother for never, ever inserting even a shred of negativity onto my dreams and for defending me to any sibling, teacher, or friend who said otherwise.

But, still, the world is a cruel and brutal place. Adversity, bad-intentioned people, and unfortunate incidents happen to every one of us every single day of our lives. Most of us get worn down. So we hunker down into the same, monotonous job because we've set ourselves up for few options. Sure, we have a large car payment, a bigger house than we'll ever need, and a desire to buy too much "stuff"…to the point that we're living well beyond our means. That's when our dreams certainly do fly out of our reach. We blame society, luck, fortune, the stock market, and an idiotic boss for our lack of professional success. We go home to sit on our porch and wonder how great things might have turned out if we'd just caught a few more breaks. If a few things out of our control had just gone a different way, we say to ourselves, "Then I sure would be living it up."

But to repeat: that's not how life goes. You make your own luck, and nobody else is going to make it for you. It's unlikely that anyone will pave your way for success. You have to start ignoring the people who say, "You can't do that." Mom was right to defend me when people kept telling me that being a professional athlete in three sports was a stupid pipedream. Even if she knew it was impossible, she also knew that as an eight-year-old boy I had a right to dream. She knew that if I wanted to believe my professional success was going to happen and that I was going to make it happen, nobody on the entire planet had the right to tell me otherwise.

If you see me interact with fellow runners, you know I never tell any of them that their goals and plans aren't going to happen. They have a right to have whatever that goal is and to try to make it happen.

The first marathon I ever ran was in Eugene, Oregon, in May of 2009. I was riding the shuttle bus back to a drop-off point, and as I sat there, exhausted and in a glob of my own nasty sweat, I started chatting with a girl across the aisle. As it turned out, she hadn't even been able to run a quarter mile eighteen months prior to race day. She'd started running on a track and hadn't been able make it around one single lap before she just got too exhausted and had to walk. But she had told her family that one day she was going to run a marathon. Her family had laughed at her. What jerks. She set out to prove them wrong. And with a time of 3:04 on that day, she qualified for Boston, a time that would have qualified her as a man because women are permitted thirty more minutes than men are. Did she ever prove them wrong! When I asked her if she held a grudge against her family for their lack of belief in her, she answered no—life is too short and grudges aren't worth it. How refreshing.

Our conversation on the bus reminded me of when I was eight and Mom had said I could do anything I wanted to. Today, more than two decades later, I still can't put into words (or type) how much her support meant back then and how much it means to me now.

The best I can do is to return the favor. Mom's a runner, too. She's gotten a few more years on her since I was a kid, and while she's completed a couple half marathons, she isn't convinced she can make the leap and run a full. She doesn't believe she can do it.

Well, I have to adamantly disagree with her. Dammit, Mom, if I could be a three-sport professional athlete, then you can run a marathon. You graduated from pharmacy school at the age of fifty-eight. That took hard work, dedication, and a belief in yourself that you could do it. She learned to believe she could succeed in pharmacy school thanks to the nudging of several key folks in her life. I'm here to tell her that if she decides she can run a full marathon, yes, she can. My pledge is that no matter whether she comes in first or last or somewhere in between, I'll be there cheering. Proud of my mom as ever.

Life lesson learned: *Dream Big.*

14

Stop Complaining

Self-awareness. I put this in the same category as being a good listener and being a good karaoke singer. A lot of people think they are good at it, but very few people actually are.

We see it every day. People driving ten miles per hour below the speed limit in the left lane on the interstate without one shred of awareness of the dozens of people passing them in a rage on the right. And we all have that friend who smacks their lips, gums, and tongue together in some orchestrated and annoying rhythm while they're eating and completely unaware of any of the noises they're making.

Self-awareness is something nearly all of us need help with. We need that friend who doesn't mind pointing out that massive piece of spinach in your teeth. Or that friend who points out when, after fifteen minutes of obvious and heavy flirting with that girl you just met, that your fly just happens to be open. My friends are the type, of course, who let whatever blunder I'm making go on for awhile before pointing it out so as to maximize their level of entertainment and my level of embarrassment.

Self-awareness is one of the main reasons jobs and companies hold reviews and feedback sessions. Employees are often doing something incorrectly and don't even realize it until someone points it out.

But sometimes those nudges of self-awareness come from other sources. Sometimes they can even come from running. In my case, the biggest lesson in self-awareness I have ever received hit me (metaphorically) right in the heart during the 2017 St Jude's Memphis Marathon. The Memphis Marathon is a wonderful event that I highly recommend. It's well organized and has good crowd support. And it has a great course with a feature that, to my knowledge, no other course has. Part way through the race, it leads you through a corner of the grounds of the famous children's hospital. You take a slight turn, look up, and there it is. Some of the St Jude's kids who are not allowed outside are pasted to the windows, smiling and waving to the runners and cheering us all on. As if that's not enough of a tear jerker, you also get to see and maybe interact with a few lucky kids who are allowed to be outside and right on the course.

Running the race in 2017, I spotted one of those kids. Sitting in a wheelchair and with not a speck of hair on his head, he was watching the runners, an awestruck expression on his face. Without even thinking, I side stepped off of the street right next to him. I stopped, extended my hand and said, "Put 'er there, partner!"

He reared back in his chair and gave me the most awesome, high-spirited high five I have ever received. When he looked up at me, his face was lit up like a Christmas tree and the smile on his face made me feel like he felt he'd just met Michael Jordan. I got back on the course and continued running. I had to run the rest of the race wiping the tears from my eyes instead of the sweat from my brow.

I have written in this book that running gives you a lot of time to think. That's one of the many reasons I love it. Time for reflection. Time for deep thought. Heck—sometimes no thought at all. Just an unplug for a few miles.

During the rest of that race in Memphis, I thought a lot about that kid. I thought a lot about myself, too, and how I approach every day. I'd seen how he'd been so positive and cheerful despite how much he had to complain about.

Which brings me back to self-awareness.

Do I complain too much? I don't think I do, but who knows? Being self-aware can be very difficult, so maybe I do complain and don't even realize I'm doing it. That's why I started thinking about some of the things I complain about most often and I soon became angry and frustrated with myself. Because I had this epiphany: I understood that no matter how hard or how long I wracked my brain, there was (and still is) nothing that has ever happened in my entire life which can come even close to what that kid has to face every single day of his life. And yet my approach to a lot of days is to bitch and moan about petty, minor, inconsequential things.

The kid's approach? He was happy just to be alive. Grinning ear to ear after a simple high five from a total stranger. Ecstatic that he was able to witness one more sunrise. Because who knows if there will be breath in his lungs for tomorrow's? He has to live with the reality of cancer smacking him in the face. Every single day.

So he's happy in the moment. He's not trying to capture it on his phone so he can Snapchat or tweet it to his friends. Not taking selfies to post to Instagram. Not stuck inside a hospital room, wasting away and playing video games. Instead, he is outside, enjoying the cold sunshine on his face, breathing the fresh air into his lungs. Clapping and cheering for complete strangers.

A kid like that understands the harsh reality that life is fragile. He realizes that every day. And I struggle every day to remember, too, that life is fragile. To stop complaining and stop taking things for granted. That kid doesn't take anything for granted. And do you know why? He probably doesn't have enough time to be able to. So much about him on that cold December day is forever etched in my brain. His smile…oh, his heart-warming smile. The glow in his face. The spirited high five he was, oh, so excited to give me. But what do I remember most of all? Just his obvious gusto for life.

I'll never forget him because I strive to be more like him every day. That is at the top of my priority list. Not the next promotion. Not anything I saw online and want to buy. Nothing materialistic. The top of my priority list is to live life with the same love and gusto for it as that kid obviously had. I have periodically failed to do so, and I'm sure I will continue to periodically forget my resolution and fail to be more like that kid in the future. But my memory of him will forever remind me to strive to imitate his gusto.

He probably thought he was just giving me a high five. But he gave me so much more.

Who knew running a silly little 13.1 mile race could teach a person so much?

Life lesson learned: *Complain less. Be thankful more.* Compliment and praise more. Tell your loved ones you love them. Buy your wife flowers. Smile at strangers. Pick up the tab in a restaurant for a police officer or veteran. Take that trip you have always wanted. Hold on to friendships and let go of grudges. And so many more things I don't have room to list here.

In other words, live life with the same love and gusto as my young friend at St. Jude's. Those kids may not have much time to live, so we owe it to them to learn our own life lessons.

15

Questions Beginning Runners Often Ask

In this chapter I answer some of the more common questions beginning runners have asked me. If you want to run, these are things you'll need to know.

Is it OK to walk?

A resounding *yes!* If your choice is between running or walking or not doing anything at all, please walk. For example, many newcomers start out with some sort of run/walk combination, where they may run for two minutes, then walk for one minute.

Let me caution you that if you're in the middle of a long run or race and decide to walk for awhile, your body will start stiffening up. You'll notice that when you pick it up and start running again.

How does a beginner pick out the right shoes?

This is the part where I'm supposed to tell you to go to a running store and have an "expert" watch you run on a treadmill then pick out a pair of shoes that fits your stride. But I'm part of the minority of runners who will tell you that's not necessary. I did that when I started and found that the shoes they picked out for me weren't right for me.

So here's my best advice: go to a store that has a wide selection of shoes that are designed for running and try on six to ten different pairs. And please please please…don't pick them based on the colors! Go with the pair that feels the best on your feet. And don't be shy—ask the salesman if you can step outside and run around the parking lot to see how the shoes feel.

After that, it's going to be a whole lot of trial and error. This is because what an "expert" and a video camera see are completely uninformed about of the most important aspect of a pair of shoes: how you like the feel of them 6 miles in. Please allow plenty of break in time before you try a longer run with your new shoes.

And to all of the helpful running store employees—please don't be offended by my putting expert in quotation marks. I do that not because I think people in running stores don't know running. Far from it. But because nobody else is an expert at the most important aspect of the right shoes: you.

How do you motivate yourself to go running?

Some people give themselves a pep talk. "Just put on your shoes when you don't feel like running." Or, "Just lace up your running shoes and go from there. See how you feel." I have also heard of running groups who will exchange shoes and gear to take home. If you have someone's gear and you don't show up to run, you're actually causing a teammate to miss his/her run. Other people will post calendars all over their homes with their training plans. They mark the calendars with bright highlighters every time they finish a planned run and use a different color when they skip a run.

My best advice is to think like this: outside of an injury, never once have I gone out for a run and after a shower and a change of clothes thought to myself, "Boy, I sure wish I hadn't done that."

What's a good rate to increase weekly mileage?

The conventional wisdom and widely accepted rule is ten percent per week, which I can't say I disagree with. Just remember that everybody, and every body, is different. So just because ten percent is the widely accepted rule, that doesn't mean for sure it will work for you.

It's best to always err on the side of caution, especially if you're a beginner. If you are increasing at ten percent per week and your knee starts hurting while you're going up and down stairs, or your legs are overly fatigued, then step it back a bit. Better to increase more slowly than injure yourself and be out for a long time.

Please also remember that most coaches have been running for a long time, and in some cases are elite. In other words, they can run really really far and do so really really fast. When a person has been running far and fast for a long time, it's easy for them to assume that most other bodies are ready for more stress than they are actually ready for. Make sure you have a coach that understands you are a beginner, which means that staying healthy and simply crossing the finish line are your priorities. Not any kind of speed record. In fact, for my first full marathon my highest weekly mileage total during training was 28 miles.

If I'm training for a race with a lot of hills, should I do hill intervals to better prepare?

If you're a beginner, I don't recommend intervals or speed work of any kind. If race day is going to present you with hills, then many of your training runs should be on hills since it involves using your muscles in a different way than running on flat surface. Just do so with normal running—not with sprints or intervals. Any training you can do that most closely resembles your race day circumstances is ideal.

Please note: if you're a beginner and don't have a clue what speed work or hill intervals are, please keep it that way. Once you get a few races under your belt and decide your mind and your body are ready for the next level, then you can start looking into incorporating those things into your training. But since these questions are geared more toward beginners, I'm not even going to describe what they are. Just run at your pace for now. We can get in to more complicated training plans later.

Newcomers also shouldn't be too focused on time, and any kind of intervals and speed work is designed to make you faster. Speed work increases your likelihood for injury, and beginners tend to be much more prone to injury simply because their bodies are still in a significant adjustment period. For those of you who have a few races under your belt now and want to graduate to some speed work, I'm all for it as long as it's calculated and cautious.

Why does my training plan only have me running 22 miles before my race? Won't I need to be able to run more than 26.2 miles to be able to get that far on race day?

Short answer: *Because of race day magic!*

A 26.2 mile race is going to take a lot out of you and beat your body up pretty badly. If you do that in your training, that's bad news because it's going to take too long for your body to recover and you'll never get to your race. Or worse, what if you run too hard or too far and severely injure yourself?

The last four miles are all about guts, anyway, so once you run 20 or 22 in your training, you'll have your body prepared enough to run the full 26.2. I have even seen some plans whose longest run is only 16 miles. I don't personally recommend that, though some runners have found success with that sort of plan. For me personally, my longest run in training for a full is typically 20 miles.

What types of activities should I do for cross training?

Whatever feels right and whatever you enjoy, as long as it's non-impact (for example, jumping jacks would not be considered rest day cross training because you are causing impact on your legs and body). I used to be a huge proponent of cross training on my days off, but now I have lost some of my zest for them. I still do extensive core exercises, but there are too many to list here. You can do anything that uses just your own body as resistance and any that are not damaging to your back. (Note: before the weight training-running coach enthusiasts give me angry phone calls, please remember that this is what I find works best for my body. *Every body is different*.) My preference these days, however, is to simply rest on my days off. Given my size, my body needs rest.

I do highly recommend any kind of core training which strengthens your midsection—abs, obliques, glutes, upper legs, etc. Strengthening your core can make you faster when you're looking to shave a few seconds off. More importantly, core training is a great way to prevent injury.

If those reasons aren't motivation enough, I'm sure swimsuit season is right around the corner, too. And on the beach everyone loves to see your six-pack abs while you're drinking a six pack.

You talk a lot about not needing all the new and fancy equipment. What equipment do you recommend?

Invest in a good pair of shoes that feel right.

Other than that, the only equipment I recommend spending noticeable money on when you first start is anything that will help you get out the door and on the road. If an iPod, gym membership, or a fancy track jacket help you lace up your shoes and get out the door, then spend the money. If not, it's all fluff.

Good shoes and the open road. That's it.

And now for some complex and difficult questions.

What if I get injured?

This is maybe the trickiest question to answer because all injuries are different, all bodies are different, and giving any kind of blanket statement is essentially impossible. I will say, though I admit to not being a very good follower of this wisdom, that the earlier a medical professional can treat an injury, the faster you can get back to running. So if you're pretty certain you're really injured, or developing an injury, then the earlier you can get professional help, the better.

But this is where another tricky element comes into play: selecting which medical professional to visit. I say this with the utmost respect to the medical profession, and from the perspective of having a pharmacist for a mother, one of my sisters as a nurse, and being married to a sports chiropractor. There are some bad medical professionals out there. The medical profession is just like any other profession. There are some physicians who are quite good at what they do and some who are quite bad at what they do. Just like looking for an attorney or an accountant, the trick is finding a good one.

I also should give a bit of my background with doctors. I was twelve years old and a pretty darned good pitcher and infielder on my Babe Ruth League team. Dad was the coach. One Saturday, we had a big game against the other top league team, but I was so sick Friday night and Saturday morning, I couldn't even get out of bed. Dad's approach has always essentially been to stop whining, toughen up, get dressed and get ready to pitch. Upon my arrival at the field, I was so pale that even the umpire asked me if I should be playing. But Dad insisted I push through. I finally got back home, slept through Sunday evening, and went to the doctor's office first thing Monday morning. I had strep throat.

In other words, it takes a lot to convince me to go see any medical professional. But as I said, I have learned the hard way that if you can find the right professional, they can be invaluable.

I once had an ankle injury that knocked me out of running and persisted for five months. I finally went to a foot doctor and told him what was going on. I also told him my priority was very clear: to get back on the road where I belonged. Running. He looked at my ankle for about seventeen seconds, told me I needed to stop running, gave me a prescription for steroids, tried to sell me a $60 compression wrap (which they sell at Walgreens for $14), all the while explaining that the wrap was going to be the key to cure the injury. He charged me way too much for the visit and then tried to schedule a follow-up visit in six weeks.

I refused the compression wrap and told him no thanks on the follow-up visit.

Next? One visit to the right sports chiropractor, and what turned out to be acute tendonitis was quickly diagnosed and treated. I was running the next day.

My issue with a lot of doctors is that they take a cookie-cutter approach. They have about twelve maladies in their head and twelve specific solutions to those twelve maladies. Their priority is to fit you, no matter how much you don't fit, into one of those twelve cookie cutter maladies, collect your payment, and get you out the door. A good doctor, on the other hand, knows that every single patient and every single situation is different. Each patient needs to be treated in their own, very specific manner.

My point: there are some out-of-this-world amazing medical professionals. My sister Laurie goes to a doctor who understands it. His priority is simple: as long as he deems it healthy, his priority is to get you back on the road. But there are some equally awful doctors, so you really have to do your homework and maybe even go through some trial and error before you find the right one.

Need a good doctor? Find a seasoned runner who knows the right folks. Or go on a run with a local running club and ask them. Find a local running store and strike up a conversation with a few of the folks there. Or look online.

Find the wrong person, and increased frustration will follow. Find the right one, and they can practically work magic. It's important to remember, of course, that their magic only works when you do the homework they give you. No matter what your injury is, a good medical professional will give you instructions for exercises and activities to do when you get home. You need to be religious about following them. If the doctor's good, they have seen these types of things before and know what they are talking about. Have trust in what they tell you and follow their guidance. You won't regret it.

The last thing I'll say is that, in my experience, a good sports chiropractor is going to help more than just about anything else with most sports injuries. Chiropractors sometimes get a bad reputation, but you need to find a good one that specializes in endurance athletes. Advice such as the old "RICE" (Rest, Ice, Compression, Elevation) method or prescription steroids or anti-inflammatories are really just putting band aids on a gash. You need to focus more on treating the source of the problem, not just your symptoms. I have learned that oftentimes the source of your injury is not necessarily where the pain is located—sometimes, for example, your foot hurts but the issue is actually in your back. Good doctors understand that the medical advice along the lines of "Well you should just stop running" is going to fall on deaf ears.

How do I deal with chafing?

This is short and sweet. Chafing is going to happen. There just isn't much we can do to completely prevent it. But we can curb its effects with a few simple tricks.

For men, you need to protect your nipples. I prefer using waterproof tape, as I find it stays on for longer. Some runners just use Band Aids. I believe that there are also some sort of "nip guards" designed specifically for protecting nipples, but I have never tried them.

With women, it's not as much of an issue because (1) your nipples are tougher than ours and (2) you're almost always wearing a bra, so the moving and rubbing that irritate ours are less of a problem because yours are more secure.

Chafing under my arms or between my legs isn't an issue for me, but it is for some people. Any good running store will have a product that you roll on to these parts of your body to help with chafing. It looks like a stick of deodorant. The folks I know who have issues with chafing tend to be pretty positive about its effectiveness.

I use Vaseline *very* liberally on my feet to avoid blisters and all around my, um, under and backside to help with chafing. And when I say liberally, I mean when I think I have doused myself thoroughly, I put that much more on again. I don't usually bother with it, though, until I'm getting ready for a run of eight miles or longer.

Just keep in mind that anything you use can work really well for five or ten or even fifteen miles. But the 26.2 distance...well, you're going to chafe. Just accept it.

What should I know about nutrition?

Where to start.... I admittedly don't have a ton of knowledge to contribute to this answer because I just don't pay as much attention to nutrition as I probably should.

What and how healthily you eat also depends on what your goals are. If you're trying to lose weight, your nutrition is going to look different than if you're just trying to feed your body what it needs to run. I can break this down into a few categories:

1) Night before the race: Most people have the misconception that they really need to "carb up" the night before the race. That's why they attend the spaghetti feed put on by that race, pay their $14, and eat seven plates of pasta, thinking they are doing themselves a favor. Many organized races are huge culprits of feeding in to this fallacy.

I have found only one result of the eat-all-you-can approach: you're going to lose five to ten minutes on your race time tomorrow because you'll be spending way too much time at the port-a-potties mid-race.

My advice is to eat the way you normally eat. Eat the same type of meal you typically ate the night before your long run during your training. Then after your race, if you want to eat your weight in cheap pasta, eat your heart out. Lord knows, you've earned it!

Also important to note: if you travel for your race, don't be tempted to partake of the local cuisine the night before the race if you're not used to it. For example, if you travel to New Orleans and really want to eat a dozen oysters and a bowl of jambalaya, or if you travel to San Francisco and are excited about trying their fresh fish sushi, please don't do so the night before the race. It can wait a day.

2) Ongoing while training: Again, emphasizing that I'm not the nutrition expert, I can only draw on what I crave and what I perceive works for me. I focus on three things: protein, protein, and more protein. I always drink chocolate milk in the morning. My mid-day snacks are nuts and Greek yogurt. And I eat a ton of beef, chicken, and fish. Basically, whatever I can find that fills me full of protein.

A lot of fellow runners focus on antioxidant-rich foods, but for me personally, I just haven't ever really noticed a difference when I pile those on in my diet. What I do know is that the night after a long run, my body craves a steak, and I'm happy to oblige. Those folks who focus on other things on top of protein swear by it. Which is awesome. For some of them, it probably truly helps them succeed. For others, they probably believe antioxidants help when the actually don't. This is called the placebo effect. But that's okay, too. There is actual value in placebos.

3) Morning of the race: This needs to be what you've been eating prior to long runs in your training. Remember: nothing new on race day. Understand this needs to start early in your plan. My race morning routine is to get up about three hours before the start of the race, eat a banana and a bagel with peanut butter on it, then take a shower. I find that showering helps me wake up, and the hot water helps my muscles get warmed up. I eat another banana and another bagel with peanut butter while I'm getting dressed. The banana gives me what I need to avoid cramping, and the peanut butter and bagel stick with me for a while. What you eat is a delicate balance between making sure you have enough fuel in the tank but not having so much fuel that it makes you spend too much time running for the toilet.

4) During the race: Since I am the world's worst at mid-race eating, I can say that I'm also the world's worst at giving advice on eating mid-race. I personally don't have a need to eat at the half-marathon distance.

I only really worry about mid-race food when I get to runs that are fifteen miles or longer. Your body needs to have some sort of caloric intake, so finding a solution is a must. You need to find something. I have tried the GU packets (which, for those who don't know, is this small, foil-wrapped packet with a goo-like substance packed with calories and vitamins in it), but found that it made me puke after every long run during which I used it. I've also tried bananas but there's no practical way to carry bananas with me, and they aren't readily available at all races. I've tried orange slices and thought I had a winner until I found myself running for the toilet five times during a long run. I've tried chocolate-covered espresso beans, which actually seemed to help a lot. The issue there was hydration. Caffeine is a natural diuretic, and making my already dehydrated body even more dehydrated wasn't a good recipe.

The only thing I have found that my stomach allows are the GU blocks and/or the GU jelly beans. If you have never heard of these, look them up online or go find a local running store. I'll eat a few every five miles or so, and that does enough to get me by.

It's important to get in a habit and stick with it. Even if at Mile 5 you feel fine and don't think you need it, take what you're used to anyway. It's much easier to stay ahead than to try to play catch-up.

5) Right after the race: The shortest, best answer here is eat anything you can stomach. I have found that after running 26.2 miles I am so queasy I can't really stomach any solid foods. But it's vital to consume calories because the sooner you start consuming and processing calories, the faster healing commences.

Chocolate milk is a favorite of mine and is becoming especially popular at races. It provides good caloric and protein intake, but does not require ingesting solid foods. I have also been to cold races that have hot soup at the finish line. Again—great caloric intake not requiring you to ingest solid foods, and on a cold day the soup helps you warm up.

Again, I don't have specific advice here other than just find something you can get your body to accept. If you're so queasy at the finish line that you can't even look at food…I get it. I've been there. And if you're going to puke it up, it doesn't matter anyway. But once you think you can actually stomach solid foods, even if you don't want to, eat something. Whatever you can find.

6) The night after the race: My honest advice about eating for supper the night after the race is this: order whatever in the hell you want to. You've earned the right to eat whatever, and however much, you want to eat. But focus on protein. I have found the more protein I ingest, the better.

What about hydration?

Most hydration advice I read from the so-called experts is, quite frankly, bad. I once read a book by a very prominent runner who was adamant about his formula for how much water to consume. His directive was to drink X amount of water every Y minutes. First, that's dumb advice because aid stations along races aren't spaced by minutes. They're spaced by distance. Even if you're wearing one of those water belts, it's not going to have enough water to last you through the entire race. Second, I did a quick calculation, and his advice had me consuming somewhere around 140 ounces of water during my estimated 26.2 course time. That much liquid will have you hurling your guts out.

My approach to hydration is that it's more important to thoroughly hydrate for the weeks, days, and hours leading up to the race than it is during the race. This doesn't mean chugging eight glasses of water the morning of the race will work wonders. It means consistently and thoroughly hydrating all day long for a couple of weeks before your race.

And minimize any diuretics. Even though I don't drink coffee, I still recognize this is hard advice to hear. Nevertheless, try to avoid, or at least cut back on coffee for a couple weeks leading up to your race. The same goes for caffeinated soft drinks. And I have also been known to give up alcohol for the four weeks leading up to my race.

Now, I'm not saying mid-race hydration isn't important. In fact, it is important. But it becomes much less vital and much more manageable if you've done your homework. Concerning how to hydrate mid race, the key to remember is staying ahead of it. Even if you don't think you feel thirsty early in a race, I would still grab some water at each station and at least wet your mouth and take a few sips. My personal preference is water, as the sports drinks make my mouth sticky. But that's just a personal preference. Some people prefer to walk through water stations, as drinking from a cup of water while continuing to run is not an easy task.

If you're like me and prefer to run through water stations, the easiest way to get a drink is to grab the top of the cup and push it together so it forms a V. Then pour the water into your mouth. This will help you avoid sucking some up into your nose. And I would avoid taking huge gulps because that will take a second or two, and it will take some time for you to catch your breath, even from that minimal amount of time spent drinking instead of breathing.

Postrace hydration is also vital. While you certainly need to consume a lot of liquid, keep in mind that your body will only absorb liquids at a certain rate. So if you sit down and chug a gallon of water, it's only going to slosh around in your stomach and come right back up. It's okay to drink a hefty amount at the finish line but remember that *moderate and consistent* is the recipe for success here.

How long does it take to recover from a race?

I always say it's best to err on the side of being conservative. With the exception of very few runners, none of us are aiming for a berth in the Olympics or a Nike sponsorship. So it's all right to take a few weeks after a long race and just let your body rest.

This is another example, though, of every body being different. Some people will tell you that getting back to non-impact cross training, like yoga and cycling and stretching, will help you recover faster. That may be true for some people. But I have found that doesn't work for me. My body needs rest. I tend to take a moderate amount of over-the-counter anti-inflammatories, continue to hydrate, and avoid the gym for at least two weeks.

When I come back to the gym, I'll stick to non-impact exercises for a couple days or a week (usually cycling and stretching for me), and for my first few runs, I always stick to a treadmill. The treadmill allows me to set a slow pace, which is best at that point. It also allows me to pull the plug if my legs are feeling sluggish. If I'm on the treadmill, I don't have to be stuck outside, a mile and a half from home.

Again, just remember, when in doubt, be conservative.

16

Unwritten Rules

I'm a huge baseball fan. In the world of baseball there are a lot of unwritten rules that players, coaches, and other personnel live by. When someone violates one of these unwritten rules, they usually face repercussions...typically in the form of a 90 mph fastball pitched into their back.

Most sports and pastimes also have unwritten rules, and running is no exception. While I don't claim to have captured all of those unwritten rules, the list below is a pretty good start. A big thanks to the friends and family who helped me compile this list. These rules used to be unwritten, but now I'm writing them down.

Formerly Unwritten Written Rules of Running. Now Written.

1) Be safe from the elements, cars, and people with bad intentions.

2) There is no such thing as a good or a bad pace.

3) Never discount or put down a fellow runner's pace or distance.

4) Bragging about your own accomplishments is not allowed. Bragging about the accomplishments of other runners is, however, highly encouraged.

5) Dogs love going on runs, too.

6) A great playlist is music to your ears.

7) The glare of the sun beats the glare of a treadmill TV.

8) Don't leave home without your water bottle.

9) Crying at the finish line doesn't make you less of a person. It makes you accomplished.

10) Five plates at the buffet isn't a Thanksgiving meal. It's a Tuesday mid-morning snack.

11) Stay within a half mile of a bathroom at all times during a run.

12) Never trust a fart after mile one.

13) Being overly particular and picky about your shoes is perfectly acceptable.

14) Drinking water from a paper cup while running and breathing hard isn't any easier than it looks.

15) The encouragement of spectators means more to a runner than those spectators will ever know.

16) On that same note…as a spectator, never tell me I look great. We both know I don't look great. I look how I feel. Like shit.

17) The involvement of race volunteers means more than those volunteers will ever know.

18) Drivers can be very unpleasant to runners. Be pleasant back at them. It will piss them off.

19) Eating every forty-three minutes isn't an obsession. It is a necessity.

20) Everyone who has a positive experience wins. The only thing that impacts whether your experience was positive or not is *you*.

21) Always wave at fellow runners.

22) Throughout any race, always thank the volunteers.

23) Anyone who ever says, "The good thing about running uphill is that you get to eventually run downhill" has obviously never run downhill.

24) Somewhere, somehow, at some time, something will chafe.

25) For the guys: don't underestimate the value of Band-Aids on your nipples.

26) Running is cheaper and more fun than therapy and counseling.

27) Asphalt is easier on the knees than concrete.

28) Ugly feet are charming.

29) Toenails are overrated.

30) There is no such thing as bad weather. Only inappropriate clothing.

31) There is not much worse than waking up for an early morning run. There is nothing much better than finishing an early morning run.

32) Never run with music during a group training run.

33) Preferring to run by yourself is perfectly acceptable.

34) Don't ever wear a race shirt from a race you didn't run.

35) Don't ever wear the race shirt of the race you're running in while you're running in it. Shirts of that same race from previous years are, however, acceptable. And in fact, they're a badge of honor of sorts.

36) Always be willing to share running wisdom, tips and, stories. We're all on the same team, and you never know who you might inspire to lace up their own shoes.

37) Eliminate the words "just," "only," and "can't" from your running vocabulary.

38) Don't judge running success by your time. Judge success by how you feel.

39) Conditions change expectations.

40) Don't start too fast out of the gate. You'll regret it later in the race.

41) Always, under all circumstances, take a pre-run dump.

42) Running is difficult and painful for everyone. Even the elites.

43) Never, ever try ANYTHING new or different on race day.

44) Helping someone else succeed in their own running is more gratifying than anything you will ever do with your own running.

45) Actively mentor someone who is just getting started in their running. It will make you a better runner. And a better person.

46) Last, but certainly not least…HAVE FUN!

A Note from the Author

Readers--

Thank you so much for reading. I hope you enjoyed and learned from reading even a fraction as much as I did from writing and living through this entire journey. This is my first book, and the entire process from start to finish was incredibly challenging but even more rewarding. Kind of like running. Happy reading, and happy running.

-Josh

Josh can be reached by email at wacklerj@gmail.com
He is available for speaking engagements, book signings, or even just to chat about running.

Made in the USA
Coppell, TX
31 October 2019